AF423012

# The Doctor Within You

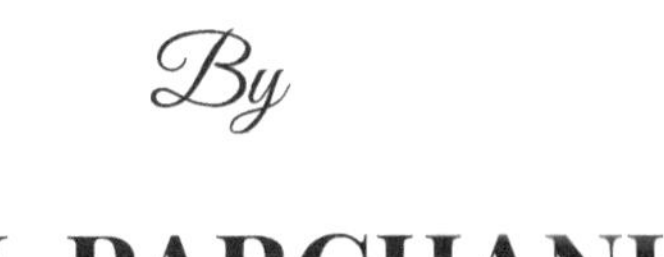

By

## ANIL PARCHANI

Title The Doctor Within You

Edition-First 2022

Copyright@ Anil Parchani 2022
Author-Anil Parchani

Published By- Self Published

Publisher's Address-G13 Jasmine, Manglam Ananda Jaipur 302029

Printers Details-JS Graphics Chaura Rasta Jaipur

Editing assistance: Dr Geeta Garwa, Bhavya Mahendra, Angel Parchani

Paperback ISBN-978-93-5620-685-4

This book is copyright, No reproduction without permission.

All rights reserved.

The information contained in this book is intended to be educational and not for diagnosis, prescription, or treatment of any health disorders or as a substitute. This information should not replace consultation with a competent healthcare professional. The content of the book is intended to be used as an adjunct to a rational and responsible programmed prescribed by a healthcare practitioner. The author and publisher are in no way liable for any misuse of the material.

# CONTENTS

# WORD OF CAUTION!!!

This book is not for everyone. Surprised? But it is true.

This book intends to alter your perspective and inspire you to embrace nature closely so that you can start living a blissful life in the bosom of nature and avoid consuming toxic medicines habitually on auto-suggestion even when they are not on prescription. It might get you in shape and restore your grooves without any unwanted impact, so read it at your own risk.

Ignoring it involves even greater risk!!!

The information in this book will cause a paradigm shift in your understanding of the naturopathic and herbal remedies that are available for almost every human ailment. Unfortunately, you may have to say goodbye to some of your pharmacy pals. Your new soul mate will be nature.

This book will awaken a ***healer within you***, allowing you to relieve all your pains and sufferings without the use of toxic medications and to treat not only your body but also your mind and soul.

Nature never betrays; Nature heals the best; Nature is the most loyal and is always (24*7) available to you. "

# DEDICATION

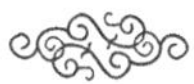

I dedicate this work to the supreme providence present around us and to my family and friends for their unconditional support, which made it possible for me to come up with this book.

A special thanks to my life partner for encouraging me to see the idea through to completion.

My vision through this book is to make people on this planet healthy with certain modifications in their lifestyle to lead a disease-free life.

# INTRODUCTION

Naturopathy, or nature cure, is the oldest type of healing system. It is called the mother of all systems. It has been touched upon in the *Vedas* as well.

Once, Lord Buddha was travelling through a forest with his followers when one of his follower monks got bitten by a snake, and the monk lost all hope of life. While Lord Buddha, who had by then acquired supreme divine knowledge of nature and its healing properties, saved his life by using smooth soil, cow dung, urine, and ash. This incident shows that curing maladies on the commands of nature is an old yet proven science. In the early days of our civilization, when modern medical science was not yet invented, there were no doctors or modern medicine. People were treated on the prospects of the blessings of nature. Nature and its sources are a privilege to us that we have forgotten in the course of time. In those days, there were some healthy spiritual customs like fasting and consuming *sattvic* food without salt, which worked like miracles on the health front. There was a ritual of worshipping five elements of human existence, like the sky, water, air, the sun, and the earth. That was the reason people led healthy lives without medications.

Naturopathy is popular not only in India but also in the other spheres of the globe. In ancient times, Germany,

Egypt, and the UK were some of the major countries where nature's cure was quite prevalent.

According to several scholars, *Dr. Vincez Preisnittz* of Germany was acclaimed as the father of modern naturopathy, while it is believed that Dr. James C. Jackson, born in 1811, was the first American to introduce Nature Cure to America. *Dr. Johnnes Schroth,* who cured the Duke of Wurttemberg in 1849 with the help of the principles of naturopathy, founded a system named after him as *Schroth Cure,* and was recognised as the greatest naturopath of all time. *I knew his system of naturopathy as Schroth Cure.*

The abovementioned illustrations are sufficient to prove that naturopathy is a science in all its rights and that it has been in practise since ages unknown. Naturopathy has been assisting humanity to establish balance with nature and its elements in the human body and harness the auto-immune properties of the human body.

Mahatma Gandhi, the Father of the Nation, was a firm believer in naturopathy and established India's first naturopathy hospital at Pune, in Maharashtra. He also wrote two books on nature titled "Cure: Key to Health" and "Diet & Diet Reform". He himself treated over 500 patients by practising nature's cure.

The government of India has also established the "Central Yoga and Nature Cure Research Council" and the National Institute of Naturopathy.

The Science of naturopathy does not require any introduction to Indians, but with modern age treatments, this great science of healing has been put on the back foot. Believe me, this science may be old, but it can still do wonders for humankind even today as it follows the basic principles of the body's *self-healing powers.*

"Belief is the fundamental ingredient of any recipe, so believe in the science of naturopathy and experience miracles with it."

This book will navigate you to the super express way to live a healthy life without any side effects of toxic medicines. The book is a practical step-by-step guide to get rid of lethal diseases, by unlocking the self-healing powers of our body.

We should be grateful to the Almighty for creating such a wonderful creature like the human body.

# ABOUT THE BOOK

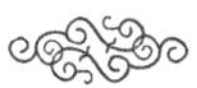

We all are unaware that there is a *Doctor Within Us*; our body has immense powers to treat all the ailments at its own, without the support of any toxic medicines. There is a concept of the body's self-healing powers. The vital force of our body is the power, that is responsible for two prime activities, The first is to conduct all the digestive functions of the body and nourish it, and the other one is to detoxify the body, scavenge all the toxic materials from the body hence keep the body healthy.

In today's digital era, where all the things are just a click away, instant things are well appreciated, we need instant gratification from things; and the same rule applies to the usage of modern medicines which relieve our pain instantly, yet they can cause several other problems with human immunity system. These modern medicines exercise hazardous side effects on human body, which may prove dangerous as they make us healthy instantly at the cost of chronic diseases in the future, as they suppress the friendly diseases.

My mission is to enlighten ten million people about this hidden doctor within us.

# About The Author

The author of this book has his roots in an extremely noble upbringing. He leads a simple life connected with his roots and observes decent ways of life among the people. He is gentle at heart, a genius by brain, and a naturalist by overall disposition.

His enthusiasm and zeal are very well known around his circle. He does not vouch for the modern medication system, nor does he recommend modern medicine. He believes in purifying the entire human immunity system by observing natural ways of treatment. He has been supporting his family, colleagues, and friends with his unquestionable expertise in natural cures. He has helped hundreds of people to cure their maladies and regain health without involving the side effects of harmful medications readily available on the market.

The same experience is being shared in utmost simplicity, with *easy-to-follow* and implement methods to treat nearly every illness with the core concept of nature's cure by utilising the power of air, water, sun, sky, and earth.

The author's goal is to change the lives of ten million people around the world by assisting them in eliminating all diseases and medications.

# TWO BEST FRIENDS

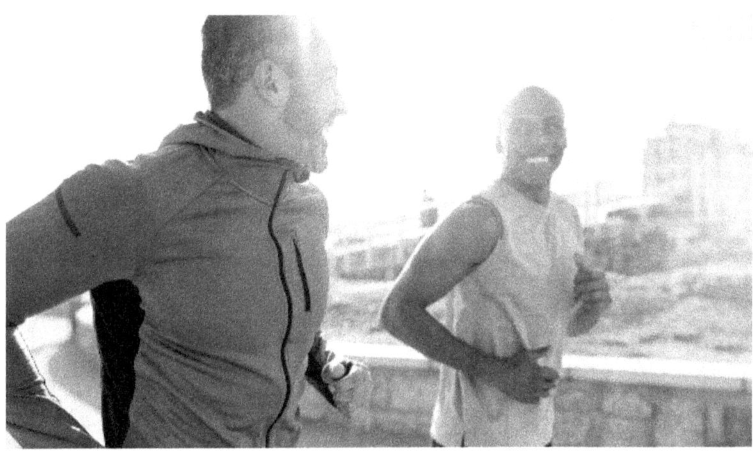

Jack and Daniel were two close friends from a small city. They received their education in same school. Both had a moderate and humble upbringing. The occupation of their parents was farming and harvesting. They used to spend most of their time together at school. They had a very close connection with nature in their daily routine which includes getting up early in the Brahma Muhurta, observing and performing yoga and deep meditation and other physical exercises to stay fit. Both Jack and Daniel maintained a healthy routine to keep themselves fit, not alone physically, but mentally as well.

Both had a dream of becoming rich and successful. They drove to a considerable distance for higher studies to fulfil their dreams and concluded their professional studies and received reasonable positions of their choice, but this time they were appointed in different enterprises and at different places. They were excited about being placed in excellent companies which would get them closer to their dreams, but they had to part ways as they were moving to diverse centres.

They were thrilled, earning more than enough to take care of their families; they maintained communication with each other, yet they could not spare time to see each other, as with almost all the corporate jobs, taking a leave is a crime but the good thing was that they were financially strengthened and shifted their parents to their respective cities.

Jack continued to work with passion and was earning a handsome salary. He shifted his family with him to the new city and was smart and efficient enough to manage the work-life harmony. He maintained a healthy lifestyle, woke up early, did meditation and yoga. He continued his good habit of fasting, which he learned in his early childhood through his parents. He was enjoying his corporate culture of partying on weekends, which made him successful in his job and sociable at his workplace.

On the contrary, Daniel didn't move his family to his city, as he was very busy and had little time to spend on himself and his family. He could not establish work-life balance; he could not handle the corporate pressure and was struggling with his health because of excessive stress. As he could not manage the things at the office, he was serving for a greater number of hours. Because of late work, he was unable to get up early, so no yoga, no exercise, and no discipline in life. He was taking lots of medication daily to cope with the ailments; a pill for sleep, a pill for stress, a pill for disruptive digestive system, a pill for blood pressure, etc. He was away from his connection with nature.

After fifteen years, a day came when Jack and Daniel met each other at their hometown for the marriage of their common relative. They had never come together before because of their busy corporate lives. They sat together for hours and recalled their childhood memories, and there were gushes of laughter and signs of joy all around.

As Jack observed, Daniel was taking a lot of pills at frequent intervals and was on a restricted diet as suggested by his doctor. On enquiring about the same, he came to know that he was suffering from many lifestyle diseases; the major cause of them was sedentary behaviour and stress.

It surprised Jack that Daniel had quit his good habits, which they both practised in their childhood, like waking up early in Brahma muhurta, yoga, exercise, and fasting.

Now Jack took charge and got his best friend out of this dreadful disease by using the tools of improvement in diet and daily routine and bringing him closer to nature again.

This book will teach you how to honour and care for your body, bringing you closer to nature and natural substances without jeopardising your corporate life. Follow Jack's example and become successful on professional, physical, and mental fronts.

Jack is the hero in this book, just like you.

# CHAPTER ONE

# BASIC CONCEPT OF NATUROPATHY

- ➢ What is Health
- ➢ Power of self-Healing
- ➢ Powers of Fasting
- ➢ Friendly Diseases

# Naturopathy's Fundamental Principles

All diseases are the sam; their causes and treatments are also the same.

- Diseases are caused by foreign materials (toxins).

- Acute illness is not a disease.

- The body's natural healing system itself is a doctor.

- Naturopathy treatment is not disease-specific; rather, it is a holistic healing process.

- Diagnosis of a disease is not required.

- Curing chronic (old and severe) diseases takes time.

- Naturopathy not only treats the body but also the mind and soul.

- Medicines reduce the effectiveness of naturopathy treatment.

- Naturopathy treatment brings old and suppressed diseases to the surface.

# What is Health?

Health is defined as a complete state of physical, mental, spiritual, and social well-being, not simply the absence of disease or infirmity.

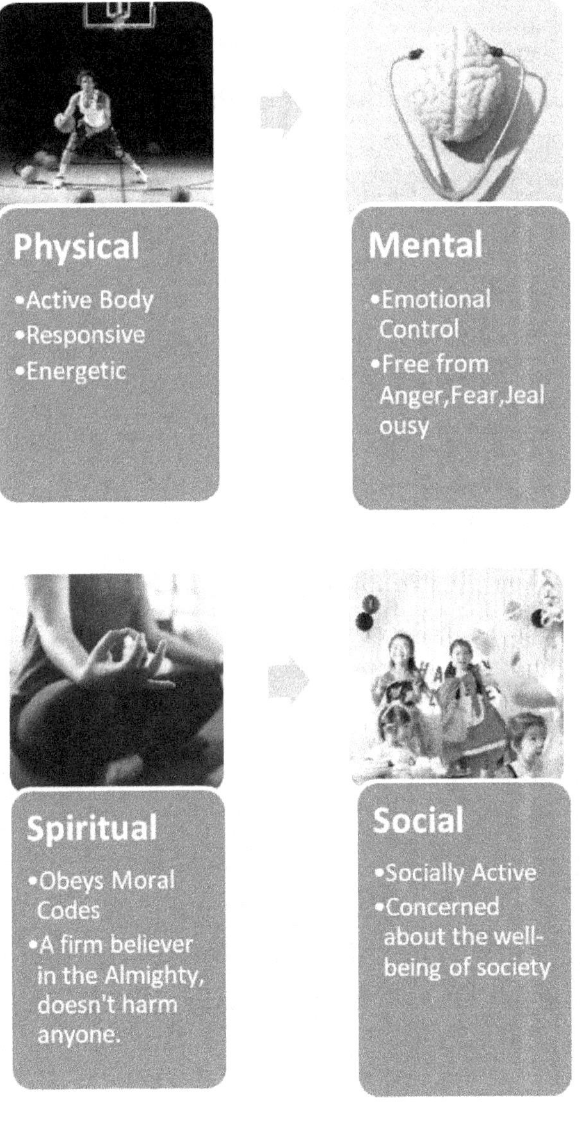

# Power of Self-Healing

**Daniel:** Good morning, Jack. Should we launch our mission of self-healing to transform into a natural and healthy life? From today onwards, you are my mentor, and I will implement all the teachings.

**Jack:** Good morning, Daniel. Sure, we will start the journey right from the beginning, as we did in our childhood. For that, one thing is required, which is belief. This is the foundation of the success of anything. If your belief system is strong enough, then you will be successful.

First, I will share the rationale why I am a firm believer in Nature's cure or *the body's self-healing* power.

Jack: Sometimes I wonder how brilliantly our bodies are created; our bodies' organs are super intelligent. They are so intelligent. They know when to act.

Let's take the illustration of the pancreas. They release insulin. When they see higher amounts of glucose in the blood, they release glucagon when the glucose levels are low in the blood. This is an intelligent system. The heart pumps blood for the entire body; the lungs take oxygen and throw $CO_2$ out of the body. While having the foodstuff, the air pipe shuts, so that food doesn't enter that pipe. I mean, this is just amazing.

Our brain can store millions of pieces of information, which cannot be imagined. It has got limitless memory power.

All these systems are intelligent, having no *CHIP* inserted nor having an internet connection. That's why I have named this "natural intelligence."

Today, the world is exploring the possibilities of artificial intelligence in every walk of life. It bothered no one about our own body system, which is natural intelligence and is working in every human being present on the planet.

## Why do we get ill?

**Daniel:** Jack, you said that our body system is super intelligent and can cure the disease on its own. Then why do we become ill?

**Jack:** I would say our body system is capable enough to cure all the ailments. It can cure even the deadliest diseases with no medicine, like cancer, asthma, high blood sugar, high blood pressure, piles, peptic ulcers, common cold and cough, thyroid, etc. But we don't allow it to do so. Surprised? Our body gives us signals that we are getting ill, and the body is working itself for a cure. The signals are fever, running nose, diarrhoea, coughing, skin rashes etc.

Now we will understand how we are stopping our body system from getting cured itself.

The answer is simple, by suppressing the above signals by taking medicines. Medicines suppress these signals, and we get instant relief at the cost of getting more dangerous diseases in the future. Instead of suppressing these diseases, we should support our body's vital energy in fighting the diseases and get healthier.

Now the point is how to support our body's vital energy, which we will understand in the coming discussions.

**"Love, respect, and care for your body."**

-Anil Parchani

**Daniel: How to support our body systems for the process of self-healing?**

**Jack:** So far, we have understood that our body sends signals that it is getting some disease and tries to overcome the same on its own.

So, as per the belief of Naturopathy, our body gets ill when toxins (foreign matter) are found in our body and our system is so intelligent that it throws them out as *sneezing, diarrhoea, fever,* etc. But when the intensity of toxins is high, we need to help our body system eliminate the toxins from the body to get rid of any disease.

Our body has a certain amount of energy which is being utilized by the body to take care of routine work like digestion, breathing, circulation of energy to cells all around the body by circulating blood, etc.

Now that same amount of energy must perform additional work of getting the toxins out of the body which becomes difficult in case of higher numbers of toxins accumulated in the body, here comes our role of supporting the body system by *FASTING* so that body's Vital energy can be preserved from the activity of digestion and can be channelized for the detoxification of the body.

This is the greatest support we can ever provide to our body. So, with fasting, the body energy concentrates on detoxification, and we get cured.

# Power of Fasting

**How to support our body systems in healing?**

**Daniel:** Jack, what are the powers of fasting? Why should it be observed?

**Jack:** How will you feel when you are about to finish your office work and ready to go home and your boss gives you another set of files to complete? You convince yourself that it is a matter of hours to maintain your position as a sincere employee when the promotions and increments are around the corner. Here is another set of surprises for you. Your boss asks you to complete the PowerPoint presentation for his upcoming meeting with the CEO of the company. Today you have no choice but to complete the task assigned and continue to work till late at night.

This happens to our body. The digestive system has just digested the heavy breakfast, given the added task of digesting the lunch fortified with butter, dal, and breads with the tadka of butter, and guess what? It is not the end of the day. The super delicious dinner is on the table, which will certainly horrify our digestive system as it has not yet finished digesting the lunch.

Now you must have understood the concept of break/rest. Why is it necessary for everyone? It is the law of nature to give the rest to increase efficiency and productivity. In the absence of breaks, we can go mad and so can our digestive system.

In India, fasting is performed for mythological beliefs. Poornima *and ekadashi* are the common days of fasting. *Navratri, Shivratri,* and *Karwa Chauth* are the festivals on which they observe fasting. The different days of fasting have been said to appease different gods or goddesses.

Like Monday fasting for Lord Shiva,

Tuesday is fasting for Lord Hanumana.

Wednesday is fasting for Lord Ganesha.

Thursday fasting for Lord Dattatray: the trio headed form of Brahma, Vishnu, and Mahesh

Friday fasting for Santoshimaa our Muslims friends also observe fasting during the month of Ramadan.

Earlier people used to fast for different reasons, but they were unknowingly being benefited in terms of health.

"FAST more frequently if you care about your body systems."

-Anil Parchani

## Definition of Fasting

**Daniel:** Jack, it seems to be complicated; it is very difficult for me to be without food for the entire day. Can you tell me about all the different types of fasting?

**Jack:** In India, fasting has been considered of extreme importance. Since ancient times, in our religious books, fasting has been regarded as a means for purification of the mind, body, and soul.

Among the believers of Jainism, the fast has a special place in their religion. Even today, they observe fasting.

The purpose of fasting is to give complete rest to the digestive system. It is only during the period of fasting that the digestive system gets to rest, as we eat two or three times daily because of which it must work. Can you imagine building a new road without halting current traffic? Of course not, in the same way we need to halt digestive activities for the cleaning of the body.

In fact, it will surprise you that fasting is a natural condition. Birds and animals require fasting sometimes, as if an animal has a greater perception about its health than a sick human being. When an animal is sick, it does not even look at its food. No matter how good it is, when we fall sick, we also have a low appetite. But we do not follow the direction of nature and continue to eat food. Fasting is a powerful way to get rid of the foreign matters. Which is the main cause of sickness.

Fasting by itself, does not give new vital force, but it removes the poison in the body which causes ill health, and the body becomes healthy. A healthy person. Who has no poisonous matter in his body, does not need to fast, but if he also fasts from time to time, he will always remain healthy.

Fasting is the best way of physical & mental purification, but someone who knows how to fast scientifically can take the full advantage of fasting only.

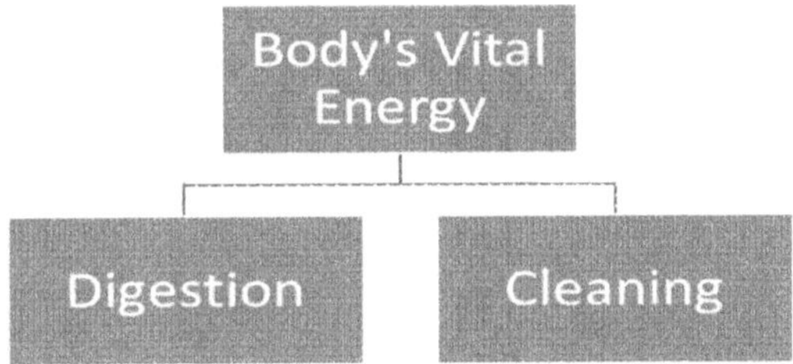


**Types of Fasting**

There are around thirteen types of *fasting,* but considering today's busy lifestyle, the four types of *fasting mentioned below* can be of great impact:

**Full Day Fasting**

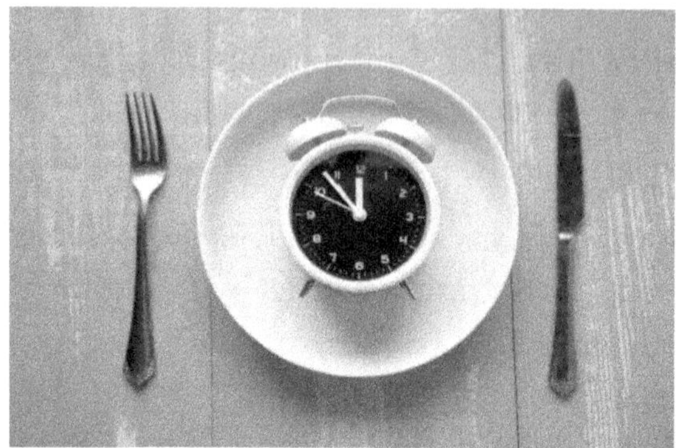

For this type of fasting, no cooked food is to be consumed for the entire day, from morning to evening. Normal water can be taken, or we can add lemon juice to water, which will cleanse the digestive system.

Remember, this is a powerful fast which will cure you faster if you are ill and will keep you healthy if you are not ill.

Recommendation: Fasting should be done at least once a week.

**Intermittent Fasting**

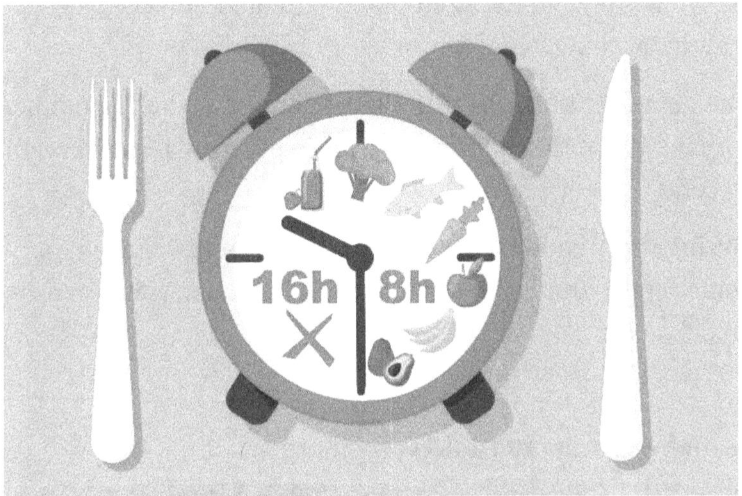

This type of fasting is gaining a lot of popularity nowadays; even in the western world it is being practiced.

This is a convenient method of fasting for those who are working professionals or self-employed because of their busy schedule, and I must admit here that it is an excellent option compared to full fasting.

*Intermittent fasting refers to a fast that is practised at regular intervals.* This is a simple yet powerful type of fasting that can clear toxins at a faster pace without being hungry for longer periods.

In this type of fasting, the gap between two meals is significant, which will give a good amount of rest to the digestive system. The gap between two meals is 14–16 hours.

In this type of fasting, cooked food can be consumed, unlike full day fasting.

For example, if we ate breakfast at 10 in the morning, then we would have lunch at around 2 p.m. and dinner at around 7 in the evening.

The next day, breakfast is to be taken around the same time, which is 10 in the morning. By this way, we will observe an effective fast of 15 hours.

During this period of the gap, no food should be taken, only water, fresh fruit juices, buttermilk, coconut water can be taken.

**Fasting on Fruits and Juices-**

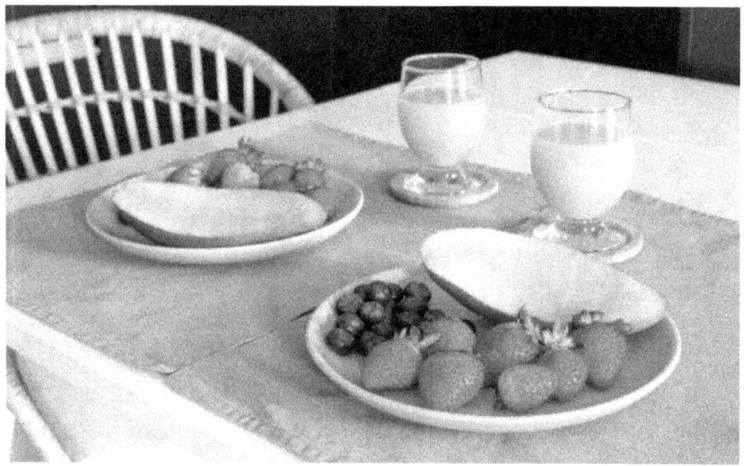

In this kind of fasting, only fruits, fresh fruit juice, or raw vegetables are consumed. This form of fasting is powerful and can cure bleeding piles in just twenty-one days.

The reason behind the fasting on fruits is that most of the fruits get digested in twenty minutes, and the vital force of the body can concentrate on curing the illness of the body.

So, I recommend that if one is ill, then he or she should consume fruits for a couple of days. The person will feel healthy and energetic.

**Fasting on Buttermilk only**

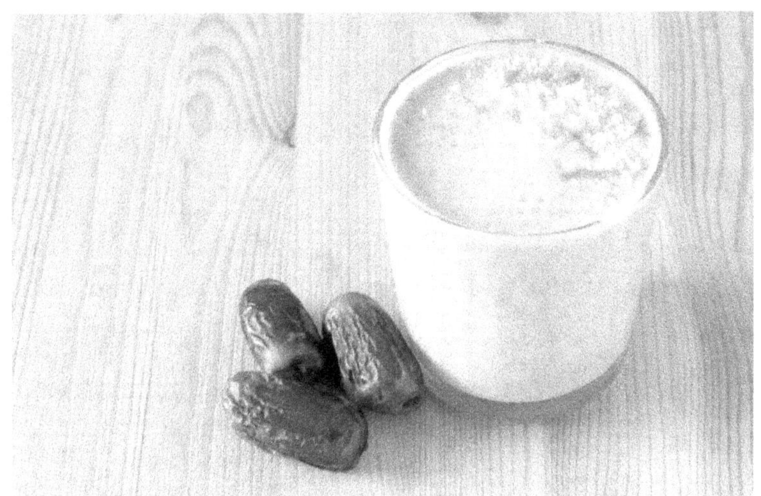

For this type of fasting, one must take only buttermilk for the entire day, provided buttermilk is fresh. The patient must consume only buttermilk for breakfast, lunch, and dinner.

If you are suffering from severe indigestion, constipation, acidity, *GERD*, or have ulcers, you should perform this kind of fasting more frequently.

**Precautions to be taken while fasting**

1.  Patients should regularly consume water, which will prevent the intestines from becoming dry and causing more discomfort.

2. A day before the fasting day, light food should be consumed so that the body's system can easily get accustomed to it.

3. If you are on intermittent fasting, avoid having heavy meals; less oily food is preferred.

4. We should avoid heavy exercise. A light workout can be done, and walking should be preferred during fasting.

5. One should take a bath on the day of fasting.

**How to end fasting?**

**Daniel**: I think it will be fun to end the fasting. After a long wait, you can enjoy a lot of delicious food, and you can have pizza and a burger.

**Jack**-No, Daniel, ending the fast is more important and difficult than starting one.

- During fasting, the digestive system becomes weak, so we should handle it with the utmost care by taking small quantities of food.

- The food should be light and should be easily digested, like Dalia, khichdi, and fruits.

- The best way to end a fast is to have coconut water before having a full meal, which nourishes the digestive system.

**Remedial Benefits of Fasting**

- A Strong Digestive System

- Reduces Acidity

- Reduces Heartburn

- It improves liver function.

- Aids in the treatment of diabetes by increasing insulin sensitivity.

- Helpful in GOUT as it reduces uric acid levels.

- Regulates blood pressure by scavenging free radicals.

- Loss of Weight

- Varicose Veins Treatment

- Joint pain is reduced.

- Heals Cancer

- Heals Ulcers

- Fasting Improves Hunger

- Fasting improves your brain function.

- Fasting helps clear skin and prevent acne.

- Fasting delays aging and keeps you younger.

- Thyroid function is improved.

# Friendly Diseases

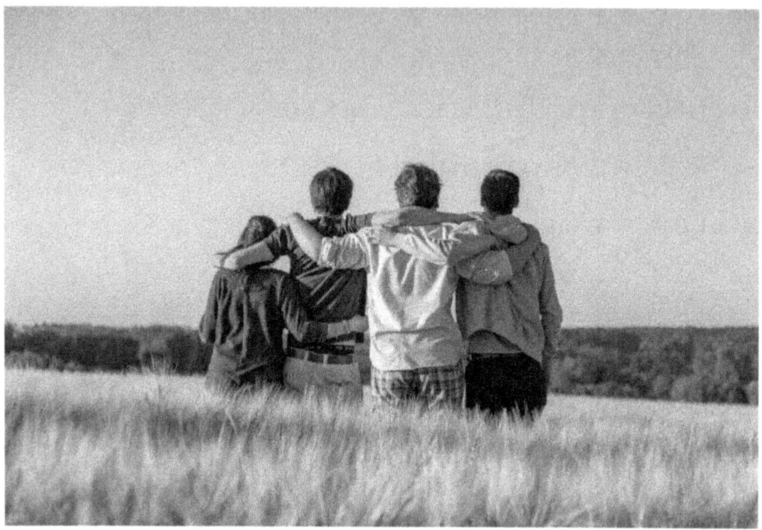

**Jack-**Today we will talk about "friendly disease" and understand the concept thoroughly.

**Daniel-**laugh, can there be a disease friend of ours? Sounds interesting

As per Naturopathy, a few diseases are categorised as "friendly diseases". As per naturopathy belief, the human body has got its own healing power and whenever some foreign body enters the body, the self-healing mechanism tries to get rid of the same and the mild symptoms of foreign body entering the body are

*Fever, Cough, Sneezing, Diarrhoea, Vomiting, Skin Rashes*

These symptoms are a sign of relief for us, as we are assured that our body's immune system is fighting with the enemy (foreign body-cause of disease).

These symptoms should not be suppressed by taking medicines that will take these acute diseases into the chronic stages where they develop into other dreaded diseases in the body.

These are friendly diseases because they tell us that the body has been attacked by some foreign body toxins and the body is trying to get rid of them on its own. We should help our body by fasting or taking a healthy diet so that the body is safeguarding itself from getting the disease in the advanced or chronic stage.

Please do not suppress these friendly symptoms by taking medicines. The natural healing process takes 3-5 days to get these under control.

**The Major Lifestyle changes required during this period.**

If you are suffering from any of the above symptoms, the following points will play a vital role in controlling the acute diseases.

- Avoid eating cooked food during this period.

- Try to observe fasting as the body's vital energy will be utilised on scavenging these symptoms only, thus faster recovery can be achieved.

- The use of fresh fruit juice will help the body get rid of the toxins.

- If it is difficult to observe a fast, taking only fresh fruits during the entire day will consume less of the body's vital energy as the digestion process of fruits is way faster than cooked food.

- Rest for faster recovery.

- Drink plenty of water during the period of these symptoms, which will help in faster detoxification.

- Avoid heavy and fast food, which is difficult to digest and takes more time for the activity of digestion to be completed.

- Don't take any medicines which will suppress the symptoms, and the chances of reoccurrence and getting the disease chronic will be much higher.

- Have faith in the body self-healing power.

- Prayer and positive affirmations can do wonders in these adverse situations.

# CHAPTER TWO

# POWERS OF NATURE

- ➢ Wonderful Water
- ➢ Balloon Breathing
- ➢ Sun-The Superpower
- ➢ Mud-The Mother Earth
- ➢ Barefoot Walking

# Powers of Nature

**Jack:** Mother Nature has blessed us with so many natural substances that we don't need anything artificial to cure our bodies. Our body is composed of five elements.

We become ill in the case of an imbalance of any of those substances. These are below described.

*Sky, Earth, Sun, Air, Water.*

We will focus on these elements.

The sky element is represented by fasting, which has been discussed in a separate chapter.

# Wonderful Water

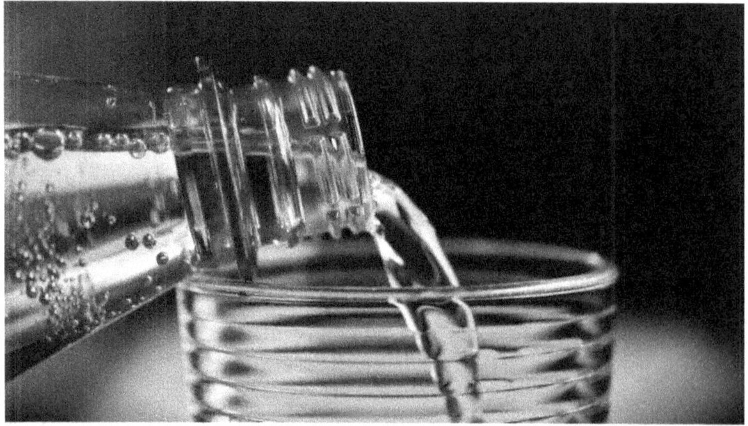

**Daniel:** Is there a better way to clean our bodies, and is there a natural pain reliever?

**Jack:** Yes, there is a super drink provided by *"Mother Nature"*, which not only detoxifies our bodies but also keeps our bodies away from foreign toxins and works as an instant pain reliever.

According to Vedic Literature, *"Apsosomoadraveednt, Vishwavani Bheshajsomne."*

Meaning, the creator of the universe has said that water has all the medicines in it.

According to Atharv Veda, *"Apsva Santaramtamp soobheshajam."*

Water is nectar and water is medicine.

70% of a human body is composed of water. Water is expelled out as stool, urine, and sweat. An average adult man expels 50 cc of water as respiration, 500 cc as perspiration, and 2500 cc as excretion every day. Hence, to maintain a balance of fluids in the body, it is important to consume an optimum amount of clean water every day.

**Water** is one of the most important elements in *Panchmahabhuta.* **Water** is life, water is energy, and water is the most powerful energy drink, even more powerful than all the so-called modern energy drinks available on the market. **Water** can improve health. We can achieve a younger and longer life. **Water** is an essential element for humans. **Water** is a profound medicine.

**Do you know water is a *powerful painkiller*?**

If you are suffering from a headache, take a glass of warm water, sip it. You will feel your pain vanishing away. Water works better than any painkiller available on the market.

***Japanese Water Healing Technique***

**Daniel**: What is new in this? We are drinking water regularly.

**Jack**: Yes, Daniel, you are right. We take water, but there is a specific way of drinking the same that offers remedial benefits for almost all the ailments.

The treatment: as per ***Japanese water technique***, drink 4-5 glasses on an empty stomach in the morning before brushing, take nothing for an hour. The water should be at room temperature.

The Advantages of ***Water Therapy***:

- Drinking water in the morning will make your body energetic.

- It helps the digestive system.

- It keeps you hydrated.

- helps with optimum brain function.

- reduces headache.

- It reduces constipation.

- It removes kidney stones.

- It keeps your skin nourished and shiny.

- It cleanses the entire digestive system.

- Excrete toxins to keep you healthy.

- reduces the chances of urinary tract infections.

- STDs (Sexually Transmitted Diseases) are reduced.

- Cures cancer.

- helps in renal (kidney) disorders.

- It expels uric acid.

- It nourishes the skin.

- It improves sinusitis conditions.

- provides strength.

- It acts as an antiseptic.

- It is an excellent expectorant.

- It provides agility.

**Daniel**: This is a superb and easy method to keep our bodies healthy, but for how long should we continue this practice?

**Jack**: This practise should be continued if you want to be healthy. It should be done daily as there is no side effect to this practice. Even people who are healthy and free of disease should practise this to stay healthy.

So far, we have understood the importance of water as a medicine. Now we will have a look at the importance of water at different temperatures.

**The effects of hot water**

Hot water baths provide relief from *coughing, colds, insomnia, high blood pressure, unconsciousness, asthma,* etc. It is very beneficial for women with irregular *menstrual cycles.*

Hot water baths cleanse the body, they ease muscle stiffness, and they get rid of fatigue quickly. But it slows down the nervous system and, hence, makes the body lethargic and slows the process of digestion. That is the reason that hot water bathing is not advised regularly. We should not take it more than twice a week.

*Hot water should not be poured on the head. It can hamper vision and slow brain activity.*

## The effects of cold water

Our skin shrinks when it comes into contact with cold water and blood vessels settle deeper. But after some time, as a reaction to this, more blood circulates in the area to fill the gap. That is why we feel hot after a cold bath as blood circulation improves. And we feel even better if we rub the body with a soft towel prior to bathing.

## Effects of Normal Water

It is important to take a bath with normal temperature water. Before taking a bath, the body should be massaged with oil. This will make the nervous system strong, increase the blood circulation in different parts of the body, and expel toxins from the body. The skin becomes softer, reversing the signs of aging.

The best time to take a bath is early in the morning. In summer, bathing can be taken twice or thrice.

According to **Adolf Just,** we should put the water on our pelvic region for the first 5 minutes of the bath and then let the waterfall on the back and the spine, followed by the rest of the body for maximum benefits of the bath.

# Balloon Breathing

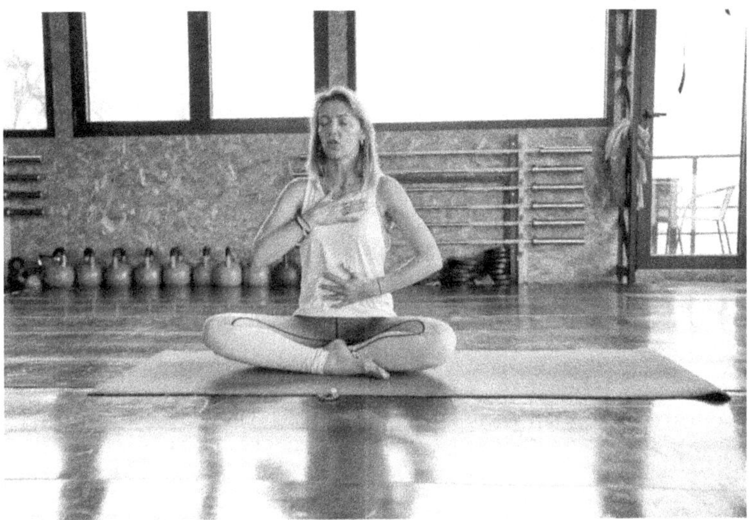

One day, Jack and Daniel planned to take their kids to the nearby amusement park so that they could get well acquainted with themselves, as they seldom see each other. While entering the park, there was an old man selling colourful balloons. They fascinated the kids with the colours and demanded the same. Jack fulfilled the demand.

While observing the balloons, Jack was reminded of the concept of a special breathing pattern and told Daniel about the same while the kids were playing in the garden.

**Jack**: As we know that air is an important element of our body, which we call Pranvayu (Air for Life), it becomes essential for all of us to breathe correctly to get maximum benefits out of breathing.

Normally, when we *breathe in*, the stomach gets in and while *breathing out*, the stomach gets inflated, which is not the correct way of breathing.

You must have noticed that when you blow the balloon, it gets inflated as the air enters it. In the same way, as we breathe in, the supply of oxygen increases in the body and the stomach should inflate and the chest should remain as is. While you breathe out, the stomach gets into the normal position. This type of breathing is called abdominal breathing, or we can say this **balloon breathing**.

**'Breathe in through the nose and breathe out through the mouth.'**

Initially, it will be difficult to perform the balloon breathing, but with practice, you can perform it well. In the beginning, you can keep one hand on the stomach and another on the chest so that you can observe the right movement of the stomach.

One easier way to get this practise is to lie down and start balloon breathing. With lots of practice, you can perform this while sitting as well.

**Benefits of Balloon Breathing**

- Balloon breathing is the best way to get rid of stress immediately. You can do this even while attending a meeting or conference.
- It relaxes your body stiffness instantly.
- It drastically improves the blood oxygen levels, which improves the nervous system and functioning of the body.

- This breathing technique is quite helpful to reduce your thoughts so you can meditate easily. All the meditation instructors suggest this before starting meditation.
- Reduces Blood Pressure.
- Through this kind of breathing pattern, all your parts of the digestive system and respiratory system get exercised, which improves digestion.
- It improves core strength.
- It reduces nasal congestion.
- It reduces the attacks of asthma.
- promotes deep sleep. Balloon breathing can be performed before sleep.

**"Your body gives you so much; don't put it to the test."**

-Anil Parchani

# Sun-The Superpower

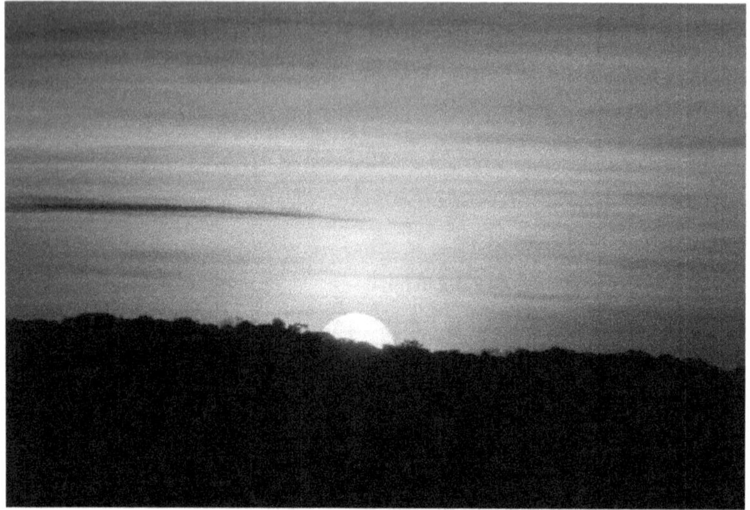

"Whose light that has no substitute for the universe is called the Sun." The entire universe gets its energy from the Sun. Sunlight has not only its *positive effect* on the outer surface of the body, but it also enters through the skin, percolates, and improves blood circulation, providing energy to the cells.

The sun and living beings have a close connection. The sun is as important as air for life. Life depends on the sun directly. The rising and setting sun destroys the germs of the earth with its rays, as described in the *Atharva Veda*.

**Importance of Sunlight in Daily Life-**

- Sunlight enhances the nervous system.

- It strengthens the digestive system.

- strengthens the excretory system.

- Enhances blood circulation

- It purifies and makes the blood warm.

- It strengthens the muscles.

- Hardens the bones

- It maintains hormonal balance.

- Sunlight endows wisdom.

- Sunlight endows beauty

- increases calcium, phosphorus, and iron levels in the blood.

Now it is important to understand how we can use the sunrays to treat various diseases.

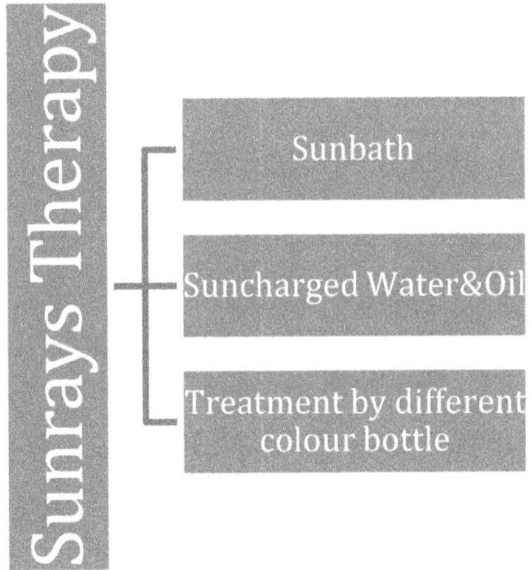


*Sunbath therapy* is very useful and important for the existence of humankind. We depend on the sun for food and health. Different diseases are treated differently by using sunlight. Sunbath has been very beneficial in treating various dreaded diseases since ancient times. With the help of sunbath, toxins are expelled as sweat. You feel energetic and healthy after sunbathing. The following are some important sunbathing guidelines to follow.

According to *Dr. Kunhe*, the patient is asked to lie down in the sun wearing nothing more than underpants. The body, from head to navel, is covered with wet clothes. The place should not be windy. This bath can take from **30 to 90 minutes**. If the patient doesn't sweat, the duration can be extended; if the sun is intense, the duration can be shortened. One must take a bath with cold water or wipe the body with a wet towel after a sunbath to get the toxins out of the body. If the patient feels cold after a bath, he should take a walk to keep the body warm.

- It should be an isolated place where there is direct sunlight and no wind.

- The place should be neat and clean.

- should be done after a bowel movement.

- It should be done by 9 a.m.

- In summer, a sunbath of 10-15 min. is enough.

- In winter, it should be 20-25 min.

- It is advisable to do *Surya Namaskar* and take a sunbath.

- Vitamin D is synthesised only when sunlight falls on the skin.

- It should be done with the fewest clothes on the body.

- Patients should drink a lot of water before a sunbath, especially in the summer.

- A wet cloth must be kept on the head.

**Benefits of Sunbath**

- Sunbath has a positive impact on your health.
- It fortifies our muscles and strengthens them.
- It strengthens the central nervous system.
- It also improves digestion.
- It activates the spleen, liver, and pancreas.
- It helps in releasing an adequate amount of digestive juice.
- Blood circulation gets better in sunlight.
- Sunlight protects the body from skin diseases.
- Sunlight reduces the occurrence of anemia.
- Vitamin-D is produced under the sun.
- Sunlight helps to reduce the occurrence of colds and coughs.
- Sunlight is helpful to slow down the thyroid.
- TB patients are advised to have a sunbath or sit under the sun for at least 10 minutes daily.

**Precautions**

- should not be done after 9 a.m. in the summer.
- should drink an ample amount of water in the summer.
- One should not forget to keep a wet cloth on their heads.
- If one feels uncomfortable, then it should be abandoned immediately. Take a cold-water shower.
- Patients with skin allergies or sunburn should avoid sunbathing.

**Sun charged water and oil**

The water kept in glass bottle of certain colours for a certain period fetches the beneficial qualities of sunrays, thus provides remedial benefits.

**Material required**

- Glass bottle

- Wooden plank

**Method:** Two-third of a glass bottle of the colour that is needed for the therapy, to be filled with water and tightly secured with cork and to be kept under sunlight on wooden plank. The bottle should be kept for six hours and to be brought inside in the evening. After sun charging the water, no other artificial light should fall on the bottle. The bottle should always be kept on the wooden plank and should not be encountered with any other metal. This sun charged water should not be exposed to rain. It should be kept away from any artificial light from electricity.

**Sun Charged Oil**

The method of charging oil is same as of water, but oil takes 40 days to be charged under the sun. It should be kept daily in the morning under the sun and to be removed in the evening for 40 days. To be kept away from any other artificial light.

# Powers of Colours

Which colour bottle to be used – Chromo therapy can be done with 3 colours, Orange, Green and Blue.

These have different characteristics and can be used for different diseases.

| Colour | Properties | Benefits | Precautions |
| --- | --- | --- | --- |
| Orange | This colour is very energetic and arousing. It increases warmth of the body. Hence it protects the body from cough and cold. This colour increases the will power, stimulates energy, and balances the levels of iodine. | Removes laziness and body feels energetic.<br><br>Improves digestion<br><br>It gets rid of Constipation permanently, soothes gastritis.<br><br>Increases haemoglobin levels in the blood.<br><br>Removes wrinkles.<br><br>It is beneficial for nervous system.<br><br>Improves blood circulation.<br><br>Cures Acidity.<br><br>Beneficial in vomiting and nausea.<br><br>Relieves joint and shoulder pain.<br><br>Reduces high blood pressure.<br><br>Regulates menstrual cycle. | Orange colour must not be used unnecessarily.<br><br>The water from orange therapy should be consumed after 15 minutes of having food and should be consumed within 30 minutes. |

| Green | This colour is moderate in nature and is beneficial for skin disorders. It is neither cold nor hot hence it balances the heat and cold. This colour works for blood purification, keeps you happy, reduces jealously and envy. | 1) Removes toxins from the body.<br><br>2) Regulates body temperature.<br><br>3) It removes constipation and purifies the blood.<br><br>4) It is useful in skin rashes; sun burn measles and smallpox.<br><br>5) It strengthens nervous system.<br><br>6) Useful in Spine disorders.<br><br>7) Useful in mild fever.<br><br>8) Useful in Heart disease.<br><br>9) Application on head ensures sound sleep.<br><br>10) Useful in eye disorders. | Medicines made with green bottles should be consumed with empty stomach or at least 30 minutes before having meal. |
|---|---|---|---|

| Blue | This colour is cool in nature, constructive and germicidal. All the diseases occurring from excessive heat can be treated with blue charged water | 1)Treats premature greying of hair<br><br>2) Blue charged oil in beneficial in hair fall<br><br>3) All kind of throat infections can be treated | This colour treatment should not be used in paralysis, joint pain, arthritis and in cold conditions. |
|---|---|---|---|

| | or oil. It is particularly beneficial in mental disorders. | with blue charged water, can be consumed or to be gargled.<br><br>4) Blue charged water is beneficial in mouth ulcers and tonsillitis.<br><br>5)Blue charged water is useful in diarrhoea.<br><br>6)Useful in Fever.<br><br>7) Blue charged water and oil is beneficial in headache.<br><br>8) Excessive bleeding in periods can be cured with blue charged water.<br><br>9) Glycerine prepared with blue charge is useful in oral infections.<br><br>10) Blue charged water/oil promotes sound sleep. | |
|---|---|---|---|

# Mud-The Mother Earth

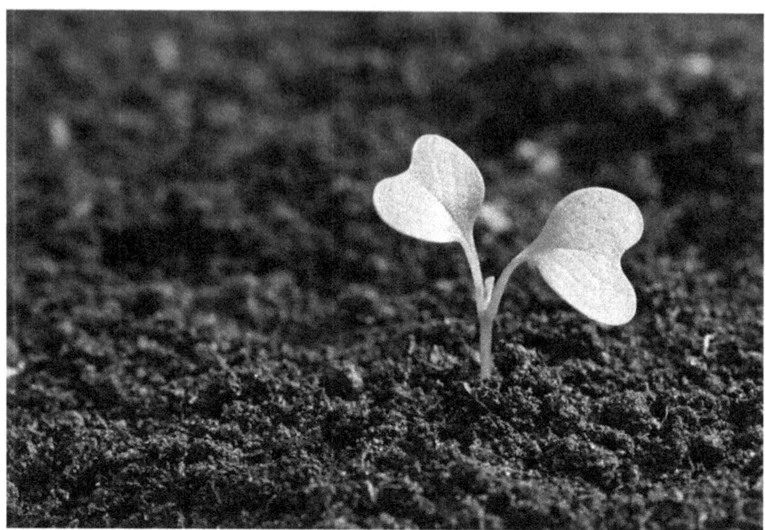

We can refer to it as *earth, mud, soil, or even our Mother Earth*. The earth is known by many different names. The Earth is so magnificent that it is referred to as the "Mother of the Universe."

We obtain everything from the earth, and, when our lives are completed, we merge with it eternally. The earth provides us with all the nutrients we require in the form of food. It provides us with all the nutrients we require to live. Mud's importance in human life is equal to that of air and water. The earth is the source of all food and life.

The soil is the foundation of everything. It is not only the mother of humans but also of all living things.

Life exists because of the mother earth.

Since ancient times, mud has been used for therapeutic purposes. It provides numerous benefits to our bodies and strengthens the earth element of the body, keeping us healthy.

**Mud properties**: There are many different types of mud that can be used for health benefits, but *Multani mitti, or clay,* which is easily available around us, can be used. Although the use of mud can be messy, it has numerous therapeutic benefits.

**Mud has the following properties:**

- **Pain reliever:** When applied to the area of pain, mud has miraculous effects. A mudpack applied to the forehead, belly, and eyes provides faster pain relief.
- **Healing Properties:** When applied moist, it heals wounds faster, but only under the supervision of a naturopath.
- **Poison Absorber-**Mud can attract poison from the body; in the case of a snake, scorpion, or honeybee bite, mud works like a charm; Gandhiji personally witnessed this.
- **Acts as a Coolant:** Because mud is cool in nature, it can absorb heat from the body in cases of heat stroke or fever. Multani mitti paste applied to the entire body will immediately attract all the body's heat.
- **It is an excellent deodorant**—mud eliminates body odour when applied to various parts of the body.
- **Detoxifying property:** Mud can absorb toxins from the body, allowing the body to heal itself.

# The benefits of Walking Barefoot on the earth, on green grass.

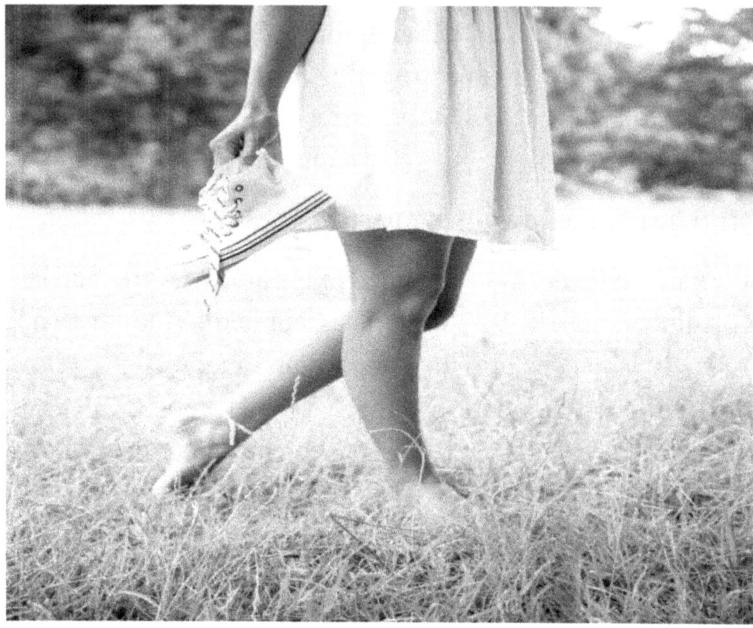

> ➤ Walking barefoot on the ground stimulates the appetite.

> ➤ Improves vision and strengthens eye muscles.

> ➤ Relieves hypertension

> ➤ It improves blood circulation.

> ➤ It gives the body energy.

> ➤ Keeps the mind calm and easy.

> ➤ Removes toxins from the body, thus keeping us healthy.

According to *Father Kneipp,* walking barefoot provides relief from migraines, throat infections, and the common cold.

Caution: Barefoot walking should not be done on the artificial surfaces of stone and concrete; it should only be done in the garden, field, or on uncovered land.

# CHAPTER THREE

# BODY DETOXIFICATION

- ➤ Body Detox Diet
- ➤ Enema

# Body Detoxification

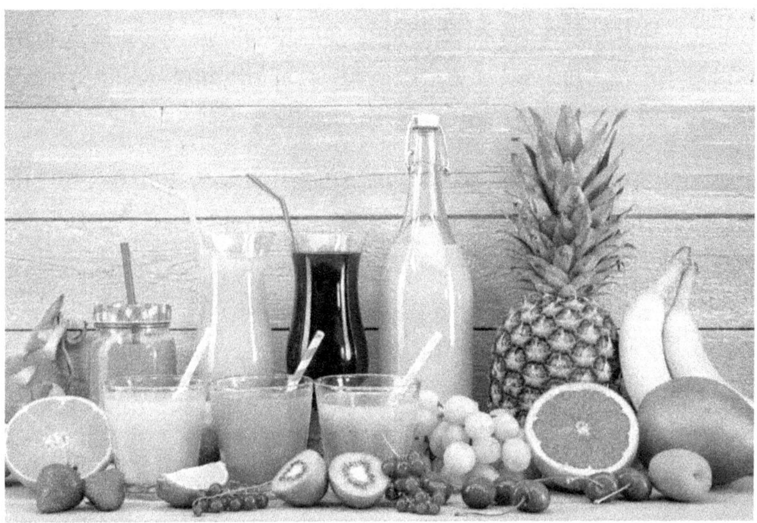

The time is 10 a.m. The phone rings, and it's Daniel calling Jack, asking if they can see each other right away because something is urgent. Jack burst out laughing and invited him to brunch.

Daniel was there in fifteen minutes. They both had a good time at brunch.

Daisy, Jack's wife, became irritated because the kitchen sink was clogged and stuffy; water was leaking from the sink; and the entire gallery had become sloppy. Jack quickly grabbed a glass of apple cider vinegar, mixed it with a tablespoon of baking soda, poured it into the sink, and the sink was washed in a matter of minutes.

Can you correlate this sterilisation action sinking into our bodies, Jack?

**Daniel:** Unlikely.

**Jack:** As the sink receives a lot of garbage and requires efficient purification, the same way our bodies consume tonnes of food material through our digestive system, it also needs to be blanked and drained on a regular basis to stay clean and bacteria free.

Body detox is an essential part of a healthy diet regime in today's digital era, where physical work has been drastically reduced in all sections of society, reducing the incidence of calorie burning and sweating, both of which aid in the elimination of toxins from the body.

To compensate for these physical activities, we must adopt a method that aids in the integration of the body's natural detoxification system. To stay healthy and keep our organs light and cholesterol-free, we should detoxify the body on a regular basis.

The following is the detox regimen that must be followed throughout the day.

7 a.m.-Detox water/curry leaf juice with lemon/tomato juice.

8:00 a.m.-Coconut water/Lauaki juice/Tori juice

10:30 a.m.-Detox water/curry leaf juice with lemon/tomato juice

**Lunch**: Green Salad, Cucumber, Tomato, Plain Coriander Chutney (No Garlic & Mirchi)

4 p.m.-Detox water/curry leaf juice with lemon/tomato juice.

5:00 p.m. -Coconut water/Lauaki juice/Toorie juice

**Dinner**-Detox water

8:30 p.m.-Watermelon

Detox water method: 2 litres of water, 1 lemon, 20 mint leaves, and 1 small ginger.

Frequency- The detox diet should be taken once a week, but it can be taken fortnightly at first.

**Amazing Benefits**

This detox method will work like magic on ill people; the toxins will be drained off at a faster pace, and for healthy individuals it will protect them from sickness. A few benefits are mentioned below.

- It relieves joint pain by excreting uric acid from the body.

- It relieves chest congestion.

- It reduces the prevalence of coughs and colds.

- It relieves pain associated with migraine.

- It relieves constipation.

- It reduces hyperacidity.

- It relieves throat infections.

- It balances blood pressure.

- It improves dental health.

- It makes you energetic by enhancing blood circulation.

- Gout (an accumulation of uric acid) is relieved.

- It helps in diminishing kidney stones.

- It relieves urinary tract infections.

- It improves digestion.

- It helps with thyroid control.

- controls blood sugar levels.

- It prevents premature greying of hair.

- It stops hair loss.

# Enema

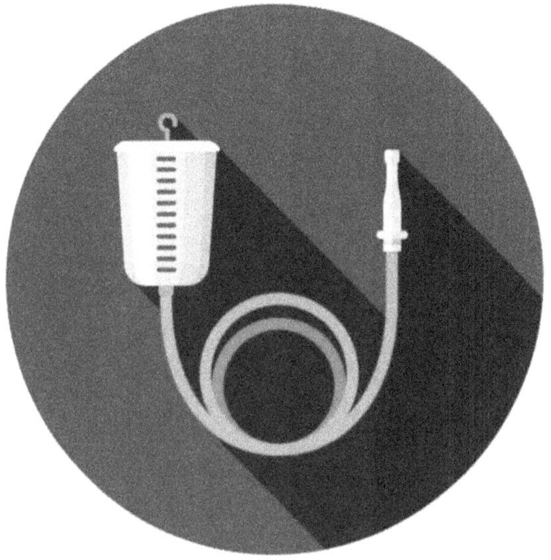

An *enema* is a method of detoxifying the intestines in which water is inserted into the intestine using gravity and an enema pot. The pot is set at a height of 3 feet above the ground. The patient should lie down on his back, insert the enema pot's syringe into the anus, and open the valve on the enema pot's pipe. The water will slowly enter the intestines. The patient must lie on his or her left side for three minutes, then straight up for three minutes, and finally on his or her right side for three minutes. Throughout the procedure, the patient must hold the water in his intestines; he may feel pressure, but he must hold it. Following the completion of the ten-minute hold, without applying any pressure, the patient must release the entire amount of water inserted. With this, the patient's intestines will become clear and all foreign, toxic waste will be expelled from the body, preventing the patient from becoming ill.

This process can be carried out for twenty-one days continuously, after which it should be performed once a week.

**Important points**

- Enema should be done on an empty stomach only.

- One should not eat anything for 30 minutes after *enemas*.

- In the case of constipation, lemon juice should be mixed with lukewarm water.

- The temperature of the enema water should be the same as the body temperature.

- The quantity of water should be 500 ml to 1 litre.

- Enema should be taken on the days of fasting.

- The quantity of water should be gradually increased.

- Enema should be taken closer to the toilet, so that in case of high pressure, the patient can go to the toilet immediately.

- Enema should be taken only after normal defection.

- After Enema, one should rest for 15 minutes.

- Before inserting the syringe of the enema pot, some water should be released in the wash basin so that air doesn't enter the body.

- Make sure to wash the syringe before and after the application.

**Benefits**

- Enema is a holistic approach for detoxification, useful for all ailments.

- The large intestine gets cleaned.

- purifies blood.

- It eases constipation.

- It increases appetite.

- It reduces headaches and migraines.

- useful in liver ailments.

- useful in nervous ailments.

- It improves skin functioning.

- reduces the unpleasant odour in the mouth

- useful in controlling high blood sugar levels.

- Thyroid control

- Useful for premature greying of hair.

- It reduces hair fall.

- It lessens the occurrence of coughs and colds.

# CHAPTER FOUR

# WET BANDAGE-A MIRACULOUS TREATMENT

- ➢ Pack on Pelvis
- ➢ Chest Pack
- ➢ Full Body Pack

# Wet bandage-Miraculous treatment

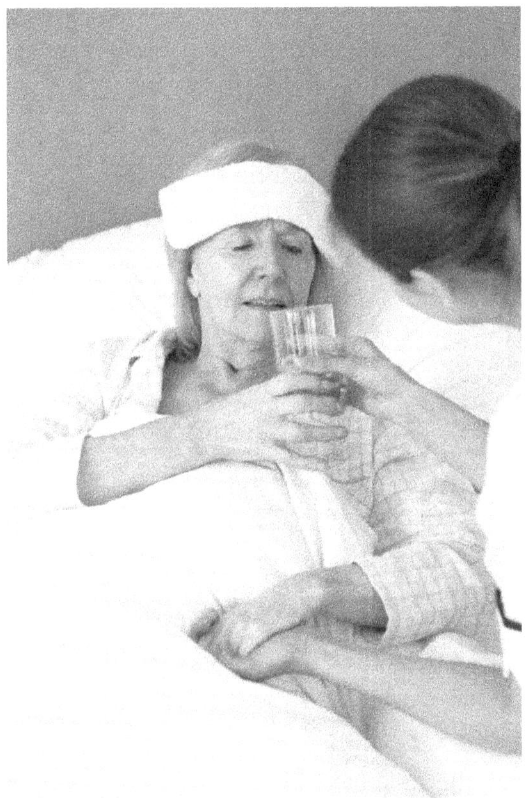

**Jack:** According to nature's cure, wet bandages are extremely important in the treatment of various ailments.

This method of treatment was also used by Mahatma Gandhi to cure his son of the dreadful disease *Kalazar.*

**Daniel-** What do you mean exactly when you say that? To treat the disease, all we need is a wet cloth. Do you think this will be accepted?

**Jack**: The science behind wet bandages is that they improve blood circulation in the affected area, remove toxins through blood circulation, and thus cure dreadful diseases without the use of harmful medications. When used to treat the following acute and chronic diseases, wet bandages have produced miraculous results:

- Pain
- Burning sensation
- Migraine
- Headache
- Cuts
- Boils
- Snake bite
- Wounds
- Constipation
- Peptic ulcers
- Hyperacidity
- High Fever
- Skin diseases
- Sleep disorder
- Cold
- Asthma
- Obesity
- Chicken Pox
- Nervous ailments
- Ear infections
- Eye infections

**Method-** To make the wet bandages, it is recommended to use *Khadi* or any cotton cloth. It's supposed to be white. This cloth should be dipped in water and squeezed. It is now time to wrap it around the affected area. Wet bandages should be applied not only to the affected area, but also to the surrounding areas.

**Pack on Pelvis**: This pack requires seven feet and eleven inches of wide cloth. We must first soak the cloth in water before squeezing it and wrapping it around our waist from the naval so that it touches our skin. To protect the moisture of the cotton cloth, we must wrap it in woollen cloth. This bandage should be worn for one to two hours at a time. It's not a bad idea to keep it overnight. This pack is beneficial for all digestive system disorders, such as *acidity, ulcers, constipation, piles, skin disorders*, and so on.

**Chest Pack-** A "chest pack" is a wet bandage wrapped around the chest. The cotton sheet should be ten to twelve feet long. To protect the moisture of the cotton cloth, we must wrap it in woollen cloth. It should be wrapped in such a way that it completely covers both the shoulders and the back. This bandage should be worn for at least forty minutes. It treats *bronchitis, asthma, colds, coughs, tuberculosis, and other illnesses.* This pack improves blood circulation and cures the disease in the affected area.

**Neck Pack:** For this pack, a **four-inch** cotton cloth should be dipped in water and squeezed thoroughly. Following that, we must wrap this cloth around the neck, followed by a woollen cloth wrapped around it. This pack should be used for forty minutes. This pack can be used to treat coughs, colds, tonsillitis, and thyroid disease.

**Leg and Feet pack:** For this pack, four feet long and four inches wide cotton cloth is needed. After dipping in the water and squeezing, wrap it around the feet and the legs till the knees. This wraps up the impure blood. It is effective for *bronchitis, pneumonia, swelling of the urinary gland, varicose veins, arthritis, joint pain, etc.* This pack is to be applied over night for faster results. If the patient cannot tolerate the cold pack, the cotton cloth should be dipped in lukewarm water.

**Full Body Pack:** This is an extremely popular treatment recommended by *Dr.Kulrajan Mukherjee.* According to him, a wet sheet pack is extremely beneficial in removing toxins from the body and strengthening the nervous system. For this, we take two litres of hot water, four to five litres of cold water, and a blanket to spread on a flat surface. Upon this blanket, a layer of cotton cloth dipped in cold water is laid; over it, in the centre of the cotton cloth, a thick towel dipped in cold water is laid. The patient is advised to lie down on the towel on his back bare bodied in such a way that his waist lies on the towel. The towel is then wrapped nicely around the waist, and the rest of the layers are also wrapped tightly around the whole body, excluding the head. He will sweat profusely if he stays in this position for forty-five minutes.

**The Benefits of this full body pack**

- Toxins are removed from the body and the blood is purified, which makes the skin beautiful.
- It reduces fat, energises the body, and tones the body.
- It increases the efficiency of the body.
- It cures constipation, gastritis, and pain from cervical and sciatica.
- Strengthening the nervous system cures paralysis.
- This is the best cure for fever.

# Chapter Five

## SUPERFOODS

- ➤ Nature's Nectar -Coconut water
- ➤ Carrot- A Superfood
- ➤ Spectacular Watermelon
- ➤ The Natural Antibiotic-Turmeric
- ➤ Castor Oil-The Natural laxative
- ➤ Onion Juice-The Panacea

# Superfoods

**Jack-** Today, we'll look at the concept of superfoods. Our own mother nature has provided us with a plethora of foods that not only nourish us but can also be used to treat a variety of disorders with no side effects.

**Daniel:** That sounds fantastic.

**Jack-** Mother Nature should be praised for creating such beautiful compositions. We will learn about their properties and how they affect the disease.

## Nature's Nectar -Coconut Water

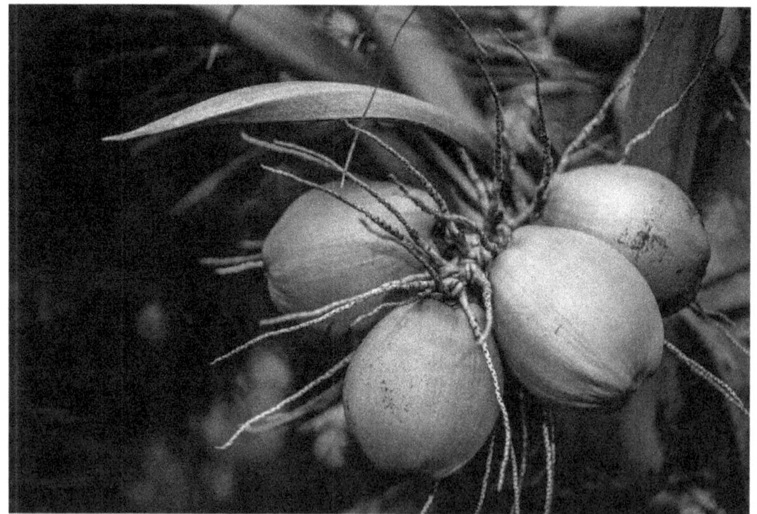

On a beautiful morning, Jack and Danial were out and about. They walked around for about 30 minutes before stopping near a garden where there were many vendors selling tea, coffee, fresh fruit juice, coconut water, and other beverages.

**Danial**: Let's start with a cup of tea. I can smell the invigorating aroma of herbs. It's very tempting.

Jack: I believe we should drink coconut water because drinking tea or coffee on an empty stomach can cause acidity and other digestive problems.

**Danial:** That means I have to stop drinking tea.

**Jack:** No, it's not like that. You can drink tea or coffee at any time of day, but not first thing in the morning on an empty stomach. I will consider the benefits of having coconut water on an empty stomach.

Nature has been so generous to humans. It has provided us with numerous tools to always keep them nourished and healthy. One of them is coconut water. Coconut water is known as Nature's nectar *(Amrit),* which means that consuming it will give you a long life.

Coconut water is the most potent drink on the planet.

Coconut water contains vitamin C, fibre, calcium, potassium, sodium, zinc, iron, folate, vitamin B, manganese, and is 90% water.

**The benefits of consuming coconut water**

- The lauric acid in coconut water increases immunity.
- increases metabolism, thus reducing weight.
- It helps the digestive system.
- reduces acidity.
- It reduces heartburn.
- An electrolyte in coconut water controls blood pressure.
- reduces UTI (Urinary Tract Infections) by increasing the volume of urine.
- reduces stress by scavenging free radicals (harmful substances).
- It provides folate during pregnancy.

- It helps to reduce kidney stones.
- Helpful for Osteoarthritis (Disease of the Bones).
- reduces skin disorders.
- controls blood sugar levels by increasing insulin secretion.
- It works as a body moisturizer.

**Daniel:** I read somewhere that diabetics should avoid drinking coconut water. Is this true?

**Jack:** That is not the case. In fact, coconut water promotes insulin secretion and lowers blood sugar levels. There are numerous other substances that should be avoided when blood sugar levels are high, such as *maida*, which has the highest *glycaemic index (increases sugar levels drastically)*. As a result, there are many things to control rather than these natural fruits, which will provide more benefits. For diabetics, the general rule is to consume coconut water on an empty stomach. We take it after meals, which inhibits absorption and can raise blood sugar levels.

# Carrot- A Superfood

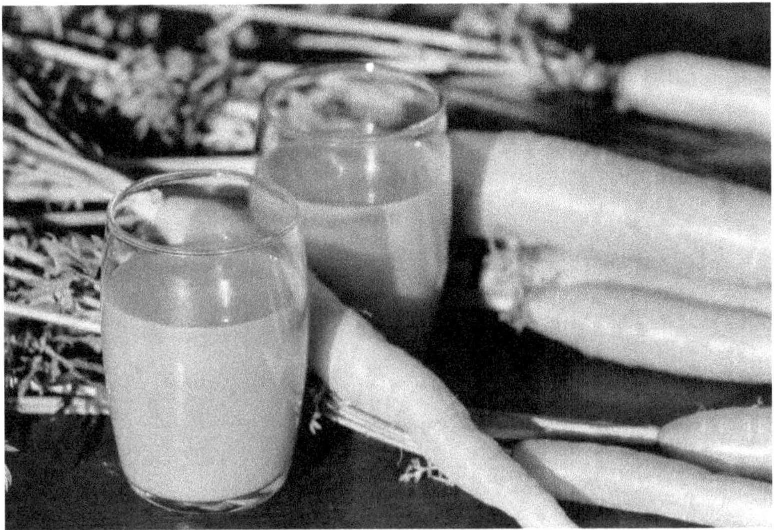

Carrots are a winter superfood. It has incredible health benefits and can be consumed either untreated or cooked.

**Types:** *Red, Yellow, and Black.*

A Carrot has **twenty times** more **Vitamin A** than cow's milk; a red carrot has **fifteen times** more Vitamin A than a yellow carrot. The black carrot is the richest in iron content.

Carrots contain *vitamins A and C, riboflavin, niacin, thiamine, iron, fibre, water, and protein.*

**Health benefits**

- Carrot juice is an excellent choice for the cure of cancer.

- Treats Eczema.

- useful for Cataracts

- It has a favorable impact on Infertility.

- It controls the menstrual cycle.

- Premature ejaculation necessitates its use.

- It aids Digestion.

- Take a mixture of carrot juice, gooseberry juice, and two spoons of honey or ten almonds every day for Brain development, body nourishment, Urinary Tract Infections, Asthma, Cancer, and Night Blindness. ·

- Carrots help with constipation.

- Carrots, when chewed, cure gum bleeding, bad breath and provide sparkling teeth

- Carrots boost immunity.

- It meets the requirement for Vitamin A.

# Spectacular Watermelon

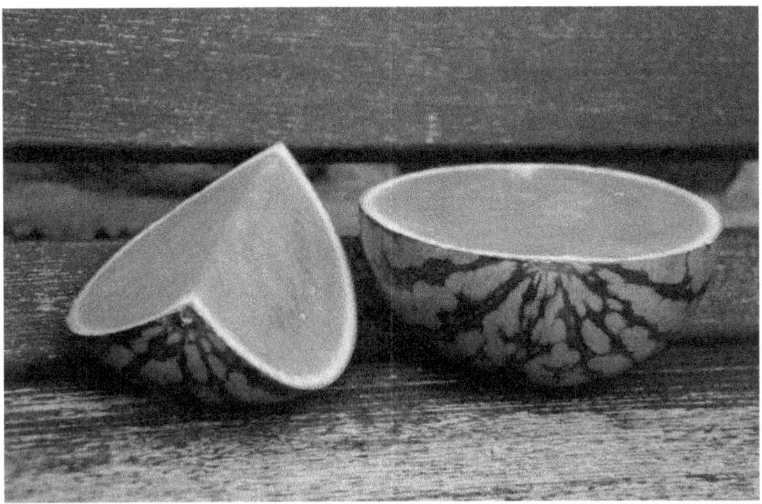

We should be grateful to Mother Nature for providing so many nutritious fruits and vegetables. They not only nourish us, but they are also seasonally appropriate. The products of the winter season are warm in nature, whereas the products of the summer season are cooler.

Watermelon is a summertime fruit. It is enriched with numerous health benefits.

*Water, calcium, carbohydrates, fibre, phosphorous, iron, vitamins B1, B2, and protein are all present.in Watermelon*

**Benefits:**

- Because it contains the most water, it is known as the "king of summer fruits."
- It contains a lot of water and potassium, which aids in detoxification of the body through urination. ·
- In hyperacidity cases, eating only watermelon for breakfast will provide dramatic relief.

- It aids in the removal of gallbladder and Urinary Tract stones.
- It is advantageous to reduce high uric acid levels.
- It is beneficial in the treatment of obesity (high weight).
- Advantageous in cases of heat stroke
- In the case of fever, throat infections, kidney swelling, and many skin infections, make the following mixture, and take it three times a day: one cup of watermelon juice, one tablespoon of gooseberry juice, and one tablespoon of honey. It will work like a miracle drink.
- It is useful for constipation.
- To be used in cases of vomiting and nausea.
- It aids in the treatment of spleen and pancreatic disorders. It will provide immediate relief when combined with buttermilk made from cow or goat milk.
- if a patient has *epilepsy, mental disorders, or insomnia,* a Watermelon shell can be placed on the patient's head for twenty minutes and will have a beneficial effect.

**Precautions to be taken while consuming Watermelon**

- It should not be consumed if it has been cut and left open for an extended period.
- We should not leave it out in the sun.
- Should be consumed before the meal
- It must not be stale.
- Water should not be consumed following the consumption of watermelon.

# The Natural Antibiotic-Turmeric

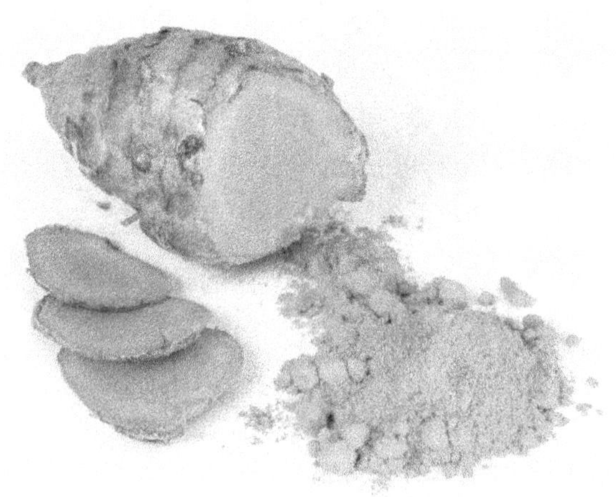

Turmeric is a common herb that is commonly used in Indian kitchens to flavour and colour dishes. It contains *curcumin* (A potent agent to cure Cancer), which helps to lower the risk of cancer. Turmeric is the most powerful herb in the world for fighting disease. It lowers the risk of infection and inflammation. Since ancient times, Ayurvedic and Chinese physicians have used it to treat a variety of diseases and ailments.

**Benefits of Turmeric**

- It lessens the occurrence of coughs and colds.
- It nourishes and glorifies the skin.
- It reduces the pain associated with arthritis.
- It reduces the chances of blood clotting.
- Beneficial effects on cancer

- It is especially useful in diabetic patients as it reduces insulin resistance and activates the pancreas.
- A report published in the journal *Bifurcates* suggests that curcumin reduces the growth of fat cells and controls obesity.
- It reduces cholesterol significantly.
- It works as a pain killer.
- It detoxifies the liver immensely.

**Side effects**

- Nausea, vomiting

- should be avoided during pregnancy.

**Consumption Method:** fresh turmeric should be grated and squeezed to obtain fresh turmeric juice; one spoon should be consumed directly, without mixing anything. It will act similarly to an *antibiotic & pain reliever*.

# Castor Oil-The Natural Laxative

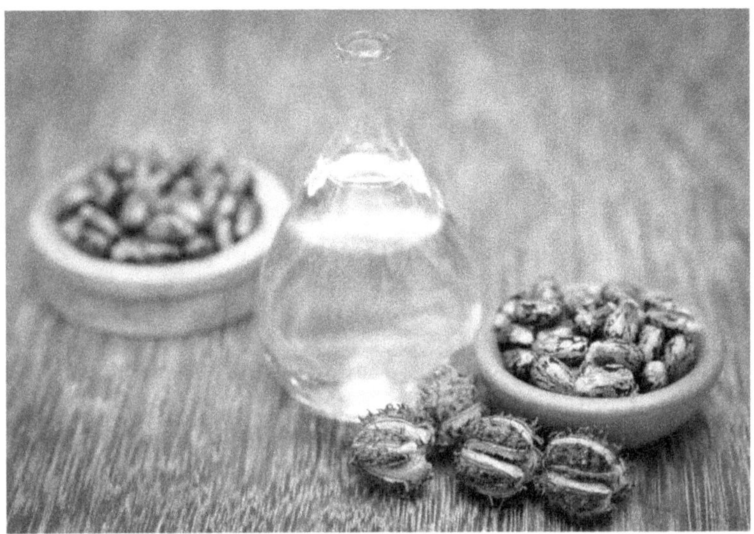

**Jack**-Castor oil is a versatile vegetable oil that has been used for thousands of years.

**Benefits of castor oil**

## 1. A potent laxative (An agent which relieves constipation)

Castor oil has been shown in studies to reduce constipation and to be safe in small amounts.

Constipation can be relieved by consuming 10 ml of castor oil mixed with hot milk at night.

## 2. Moisturising lotion (Natural)

*Ricinoleic acid*, found in castor oil, is a powerful moisturiser.

Castor oil can be used on your face and body when combined with a carrier oil such as coconut, almond, or sesame oil.

Castor oil can be used in place of artificial moisturiser to soften your skin.

## 3. Wound Healing

Castor oil creates a moist environment around the wound, which helps to keep it moist and prevents it from drying out. Furthermore, castor oil promotes tissue growth, which aids in the faster healing of wounds.

## 4. Anti-inflammatory properties

Castor oil has been shown in studies to reduce inflammation (swelling) and pain, providing relief from joint pain.

## 5. Aids in acne reduction

Castor oil contains antimicrobial properties that help to reduce bacteria, soothe skin, and treat acne.

## 6. Fungicidal properties

Castor oil has antifungal properties, according to several studies. Castor oil can be used to treat oral fungal infections. In the case of mouth ulcers, simply applying a coat of castor oil to the mouth produces excellent results.

To get rid of dandruff, mix it with almond or sesame oil and apply it to your scalp

## 7. Hair care

Castor oil functions similarly to a hair conditioner. When combined with a carrier oil such as coconut, sesame, or mustard oil, it will leave your hair silky and shiny.

 If your hair is dry, use castor oil to hydrate it.

Apply castor oil mixed with coconut or mustard oil to hair loss. Castor oil adds volume to hair and can be used to treat baldness.

## 8. Aids in Wrinkle reduction

Wrinkles can be reduced by combining castor oil and pure almond oil. For the best results, apply it to your face and leave it on overnight.

## 9. Chapped lips

Castor oil moisturizes and nourishes dry lips. This magical oil should be used in place of your current lip balm.

## 10. Sunburn

Castor oil has a soothing effect on sunburned skin. Apply to the affected skin to get relief from a burning sensation right away.

## 11. Eye Protection

Two drops should be applied to each eye. It will help to relieve stress after a long period of study or screen time. It will make your eyes feel better. Please use it only at night because it causes temporary blurring of vision, and do not walk after applying it to your eyes.

To improve vision, apply two drops of castor oil to each eye for thirty days.

**Daniel**- Is there any risk to using castor oil?

**Jack**: Yes, there are a few of them:

- Nausea and vomiting
- Loose motions
- Should not be used by pregnant women.

# Onion Juice-The Panacea

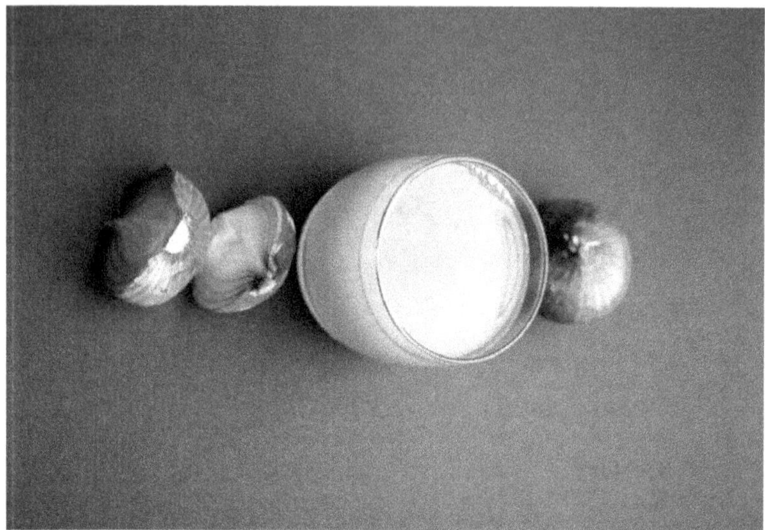

The onion is a super food which offers a variety of benefits pertaining to health. You will wonder why you have been using onions since childhood but have observed no tangible benefits.

Any food that is cooked loses its beneficial vitamins, minerals, and other substances, and there are specific ways to use onion for remedial purposes.

**The following are the remedial benefits of onion juice:**

- Weight loss
- To reduce the weight, we should take onion juice with a mixture of honey and water. Take the juice from one large onion bulb and mix it with two teaspoons of honey. We should take it on an empty stomach.
- Onion juice is helpful in relaxing airways and muscles, which provides relief from asthma symptoms.

- Onion juice is helpful in improving digestion as it supplies fibre in abundance.
- Sulphur in onion juice controls blood sugar levels.
- It gives instant relief from fever, colds, and cough.
- Onion juice cures skin infections as well.
- Keratin handles hair growth; *sulphur* in onion juice supplies amino acids which are rich in *sulphur*. Even in severe hair loss cases, onion juice is a remedial therapy.
- Onion juice reduces premature greying of hair.

**How to use Onion juice for hair care**

- Mix onion juice with Aloe Vera gel for hair fall.
- Mix onion juice with coconut oil for dry hair.
- Apply onion juice with lemon juice to dandruff. Onion
- Onion juice with almond oil for premature greying of hair
- Onion juice with castor oil for baldness or alopecia

# CHAPTER SIX

# THE SUPER INTELLIGENT DIET

- ➢ The Purpose of Intelligent Diet
- ➢ The Protocol of Intelligent Diet

# Super Intelligent Diet

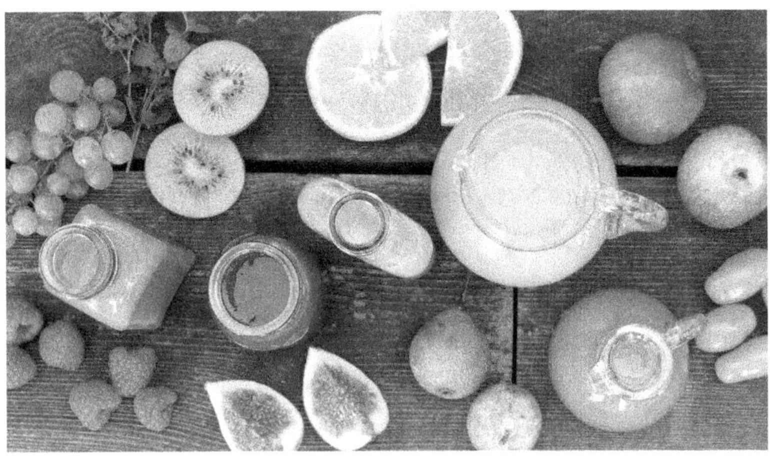

**Jack:** Today I will brief you about the super intelligent diet, which keeps us healthy and drains the toxins from our bodies, which will help us to be healthy forever.

Daniel laughs. Can a diet be intelligent?

**Jack**: Yes, why not?

We know that our body systems are super smart. They work intelligently to perform various activities to keep us alive and healthy. Besides that, they keep on detoxifying our bodies to keep them healthy. So, to integrate the smart system, our diet should also be smart to get in sync with it. But in today's digital era where food is likewise on the digital platform, we are consuming lots of pizzas, burgers, and all other junk food in the world, which disrupts the normal efficient working of the body's systems. Because of this, the detoxification of the body does not get the foreign matter out of the body and these toxins become the cause of lifestyle diseases like hypertension, diabetes, stress, and neurological disorders by making the immune system of the body weaker. We show no mercy to our digestive system and keep on consuming food enriched with high amounts of fats, spices, and artificial substances, which frighten our body system. It left us with no choice but to have these kinds of dreadful disorders.

**The Goal of the Super Intelligent Diet**

Toxins in the body are the primary cause of disease. The *Super Intelligent Diet's* goal is to help our digestive system excrete toxins from our bodies by making minor changes to our daily diet, which not only nourishes our bodies with all the required essential food groups like carbohydrates, proteins, fats, vitamins, and minerals, but also improves the digestive process, resulting in fewer toxins in the body. A healthy diet supports our body's cleansing system, which removes toxins and free radicals (harmful substances) from the body and thus keeps us disease-free.

**"Feed your body smartly,"**

-Parchani, Anil

**Protocol of *Super Intelligent Diet***

The steps to follow for the *Super Intelligent Diet*

The smart diet consists of three steps: **Breakfast, Lunch, and Dinner**. Now we'll go over each meal in detail.

**BREAKFAST:** At breakfast, we should eat fresh fruits only, based on our body weight. We'll see how this works with an example.

| Body weight (Kgs) | Qty of fruits (Gm) |
| --- | --- |
| 60 | 600 |
| 70 | 700 |
| 80 | 800 |

Bodyweight-70KG

Quantity of fruits to be taken-Body weight*10 Grams

=70*10=700 GMS

**Jack:** Today I will brief you about the super intelligent diet, which keeps us healthy and drains the toxins from our bodies, which will help us to be healthy forever.

Daniel laughs. Can a diet be intelligent?

**Jack**: Yes, why not?

So, according to the example above, the person will have 700 g of fresh fruit for breakfast.

Depending on availability or preference, you can combine three to four different types of fruits for breakfast.

**Lunch:** Lunch should be served around 1 p.m.

We'll eat two plates of lunch.

The formula is that we will have 50 percent salads and raw vegetables, and the other 50 percent will be food.

Plate one should only contain raw vegetables and salads. The amount of salad will be determined by the table below:

| Normal Diet | Super Intelligent Diet |
| --- | --- |
| 2 Chapati+ Vegetable | 1 Chapati + Vegetable + Full plate of salads |
| 4 Chapati+ Vegetable | 2 Chapati + Vegetable + Full plate of salads |
| 6 Chapati+ Vegetable | 3 Chapati + Vegetable + Full plate of salads |

In contrast to reduced Chapati consumption, salad and raw vegetable serving sizes should be sufficient to satisfy the appetite.

You can include any salad you want, such as tomato, cucumber, cabbage, spinach, carrot, and so on.

Plate two will consist of homely, cooked foods such as rice or chapati, dal, vegetables, and will be less spicy.

*Nota bene: Plate one should be eaten first.*

**Dinner**: We'll eat dinner around 7 p.m. Dinner will contain the same ingredients as Lunch, plates one and two and should be consumed as directed above.

## Precautions

- Only home-cooked food should be served on plate two; no outside food should be consumed.

- Plate one should be consumed first, no exceptions.

- Consume dry fruits if you are hungry in between diets. The maximum amount of dry fruit should not exceed the size of a fist.

**Benefits of *Super Intelligent Diet***

- Improves Digestion.

- It relieves Acidity.

- It eases Constipation.

- Detoxify your body.

- Eliminate Allergens.

- Supply fibres.

- It keeps you energetic.

- It reduces the occurrence of colds and coughs.

- It reduces joint pain by eliminating Uric acid.

- Blood pressure treatment

- Thyroid function can be restored.

- Helpful for Migraine

- It reduces joint pain.

- Makes skin gleam

- Beneficial for deep sleep

- It reduces kidney disorders.

- Helpful for improving vision

- Reduces hair loss

**Daniel:** So, Jack, how long should I keep this diet up? Can I take a break from this monotonous diet if I so desire?

**Jack:** How long do you want to be healthy for?

**Daniel:** I'm laughing. Of course, I want to be healthy for the rest of my life.

**Jack:** You have provided an answer to your question. This diet will be followed indefinitely because it has no negative side effects, but you may indulge in a cheat day once a week.

**Daniel:** Thank you so much for allowing me to have this one day (I was overjoyed to hear this).

# CHAPTER SEVEN

# CONSTIPATION-THE "MOTHER OF ALL DISORDERS"

- ➢ The Causes of Constipation
- ➢ Constipation Treatment

# Constipation-The "Mother of All Disorders"

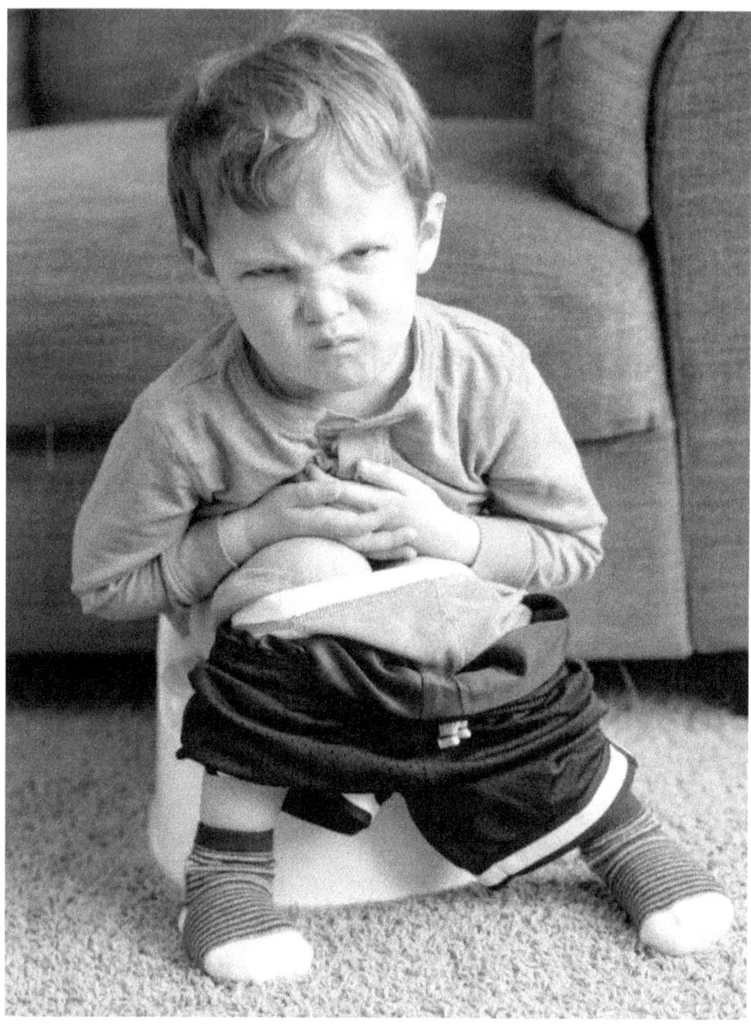

**Jack**- The foods we eat are digested by our bodies. It nourishes and energizes the entire body while also strengthening the brain. Food that has not been digested is referred to as faeces, and it is secreted from the body by the excretory system. However, full faeces are not always excreted; they remain in the large intestine and begin to rot. *Constipation* is the medical term for this condition. When this scrap remains in the body for an extended period, it ferments and emits gases that cause a variety of diseases.

When waste remains in the intestine for an extended period, it is absorbed by the intestines and enters the bloodstream. It enters the body through the blood and causes diseases such as headaches and high blood pressure. In addition to joint pain, nausea, and vomiting, the gas produced by fermentation puts pressure on the heart. When the gas reaches the stomach, it is expelled through the mouth as burps, causing tooth decay and oral diseases. That is why constipation is referred to as the "mother of all diseases."

**Daniel**-What are the reasons for Constipation?

**Jack**- Constipation can be caused by a variety of factors.

- Inadequate water intake
- Insufficient fibre intake.
- Consumption of spicy foods.
- Smoking
- Alcohol intake
- Stress
- Avoiding nature's call
- Irregular sleep
- Lethargic routine
- Overeating also causes constipation.
- Tea and coffee consumption
- Consumption of oily foods.
- Lack of fasting practice
- Consuming fewer salads
- Fresh fruits are consumed infrequently or not at all.

- Lack of exercise
- Long sitting
- Stay awake until late at night
- Not waking up early
- Having food without hunger
- Having too much fast and junk food
- There is less gap between meals.
- Overeating

**Managing Constipation**

- Have a good sleep.

- Exercise regularly.

- Have plenty of water, preferably hot water.

- At least 60% of your overall diet should be composed of salads and fruits.

- Hot water an enema is extremely beneficial for chronic constipation (for more details, please refer to the chapter on Enema).

- Apply the wet pack often. It will help to loosen the waste material accumulated in the intestine. (For more details, please refer to the chapter on Wet Packs).

- Observe fasting. It will give the body vital energy to work on detoxification. (Please refer to the chapter on fasting). *Intermittent fasting* is also extraordinarily effective in easing constipation.

- Take meals as per the protocol of a *Super Intelligent* Diet, which will supply an ample number of fibres in the body, The quality of fibres is that they absorb a lot of water, which makes stool soft and easy to pass, which will cleanse the body. (see chapter six for more information on the Super Intelligent Diet.)

- Meditation is helpful in reducing stress, which is indirectly helpful in controlling constipation.

- *The Japanese Water Technique* is also useful in controlling constipation. (Please refer to the chapter on Japanese Water Technique).

# CHAPTER EIGHT

# DIABETES MELLITUS

- ➤ Definition
- ➤ Symptoms
- ➤ Management of DM
- ➤ Natural way of controlling DM
- ➤ Diet Management
- ➤ Controlling effectively by Fasting

# Diabetes Mellitus

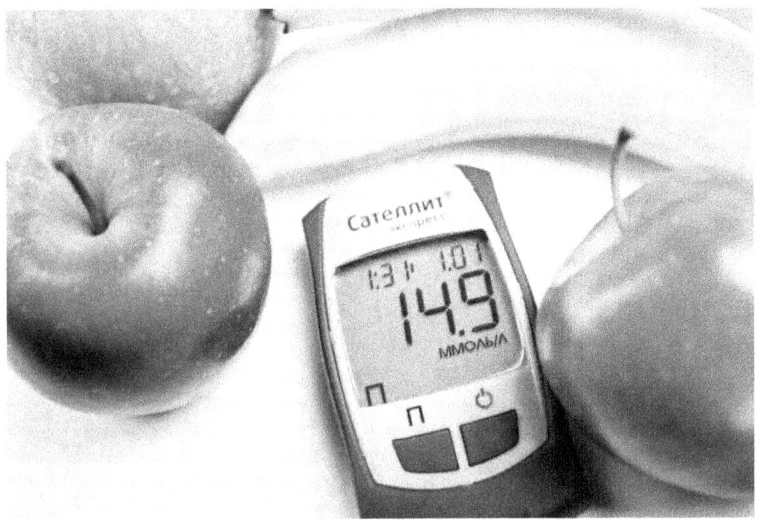

**Daniel-** What are the consequences of high blood sugar levels on the body? Is there a natural cure for this disease?

**Jack:** *"This is a pancreatic disease."*

Diabetes is characterised by abnormally high blood glucose levels. Diabetes is classified into two types: Type 1 and Type 2. There is a flaw in the manufacturing process of insulin. Insulin must be administered daily to control it. We will only discuss Type 2 diabetes here. The main cause of type 2 diabetes is a lack of insulin release, also known as insulin resistance. The following are the primary causes of DM (Diabetes Mellitus):

- Heredity

- Inadequate physical activity

- Stress

- Use of toxic medications (steroids)

**Symptoms**

- Excessive Thrust

- Excessive Urination

- Rapid weight loss

- Excessive Hunger

- Fatigue/weakness

- Blurred Vision

- Skin dryness or irritation

- Delayed wound healing

Diabetes is not a disease; it is a syndrome, which means it is a collection of diseases that can lead to a variety of complications. It can harm the kidneys, heart, eyes, and nervous system, as well as impair blood circulation, cause diabetic feet, and raise blood pressure.

**Management of DM**

Diabetes Management in Three Steps:

**1. Diet:** Diet is very important in diabetes management; the patient must be very selective in selecting a diet.

A *low-calorie* diet plan should be followed.

**2. Exercise:** 30 minutes of physical activity per day can help you control your diabetes.

**3 Detoxification**-Diabetic patients should detoxify on a regular basis to keep their bodies free of toxins and healthy.

## A natural approach to diabetes management

Mother Nature, thank you for providing some excellent substances that will aid in the natural treatment of diabetes.

**1.Ancient Power of Triphala and Fenugreek Seeds:** This is an age-old, tried-and-true formula that has been used since *ancient times*.

Both ingredients can lower high blood sugar levels, thereby controlling diabetes. One teaspoon of *Triphala* powder soaked in a glass of water overnight along with one teaspoon of *Fenugreek* seeds soaked in a separate glass of water.

Both glasses should be consumed first thing in the morning on an empty stomach. First, consume the *Triphala* powder mixture, followed by the second glass of *fenugreek* seeds to be chewed.

This medication should only be used for ninety days, by which time the symptoms should have subsided.

If the symptoms persist after ninety days, we can restart this treatment after a fifteen-day break.

**2.Powerful Karela**: Karela is a powerful herb that can help you control your diabetes. Many people consume this vegetable to reduce their DM, but some find it difficult to consume because it is bitter, so the following could be an excellent choice to get the maximum benefits of Karela without even consuming one.

Because our feet are the best parts for absorption of anything, we should soak them in Karela juice for at least two hours. Soaking the feet ensures that the substance is absorbed almost immediately, ensuring instant entry into the bloodstream and thus providing a super-quick effect.

You will feel some bitterness on your tongue while your feet soak in the Karela juice, and you will reap the full benefits of the Karela, which means you can get out of the soak. This is an excellent way to control your high blood sugar levels without causing any side effects.

Just make sure the juice is fresh and not packaged at the store.

**3. Onion Juice**: Onion juice is extremely effective at lowering blood sugar levels. On an empty stomach, consume one spoon of onion juice daily. After consuming this superfood juice, you will notice that your blood glucose levels are under control.

**Dietary Management**

Management of diabetes relies heavily on diet. Raw vegetables and fruits can help control diabetes more effectively. A Super Intelligent diet curriculum should be followed (refer to the chapter on Super Intelligent Diet). Diabetes can be reversed with this diet. It may seem unbelievable, but it is possible to reverse the symptoms of diabetes.

**Restrictions**

Sugar, salt, refined flour (Maida), potato, rice, sweet potato, meat, eggs, fish, tobacco, and alcohol are all prohibited.

**Exercise**

Exercising is just as important for diabetics as breathing. Because the body's metabolism mechanism is hampered, excess fat must be eliminated through regular exercise. The following are some ideas for fat loss. You may select any of your options.

- Walk for at least 40 minutes at a brisk pace.

- Running; cycling; swimming

**Asana**: *Jaanushirshasan, Halaasan, Mandukasana, Pawanmuktasana, Yoga Mudra*, etc.

**Pranayama**-*Kapalbhati, Bastrika, Moolbandh, Uddiyanbandh*

## Detoxification

1. Body Detox-Enema is the best thing to do in the morning on an empty stomach; it will have an immense beneficial impact on controlling diabetes. (For a detailed method of enema, please refer to the full chapter on enema). You can perform for **21 days**; later performances can be done once a week.

2. Detox Juice: It is necessary to cleanse the intestines regularly. One should consume cucumber juice daily before breakfast after performing an enema. This is a powerful detoxifying juice that will not only remove toxins from the body at a faster pace but also supply fibre and water in abundance, keeping you hydrated and nourished. This juice will work like an internal air conditioner for the body in the summer.

Method: Peel a fresh cucumber, then make the refreshing drink with a cold-pressed juicer or a mixer. You can season it with lemon to taste, but not with salt. This miracle drink should be a regular part of your diet for a long time. It has no negative side effects.

## Controlled by fasting

Fasting on a regular basis is one of the most effective ways to control diabetes. As stated in Chapter One, all diseases are caused by foreign matter in the body, and the treatment is to detoxify your body by fasting on a regular basis. If the patient is unable to fast for a full day, he can opt for intermittent fasting, which consists of fasting for *16 hours* per day and provides the same benefits as full-day fasting without the inconvenience of going without meals for a full day. Diabetes symptoms can be reversed by fasting. If your glucose levels drop while fasting, consuming jaggery will instantly restore them to normal.

The specifics of fasting are covered in the exclusive chapter. (Please refer to the chapter on Fasting.)

should be avoided if you have diabetes

- Dates
- Resins
- Alcohol
- Cold Drinks
- Oily food
- Tea
- Coffee
- Tobacco
- Meat
- Fish
- Egg
- Cake, biscuits, and breads
- Chocolate
- Potato
- White rice

# CHAPTER NINE

# THYROID

- ➢ Definition
- ➢ Reasons and symptoms
- ➢ Four Pillars of Thyroid management

# Thyroid

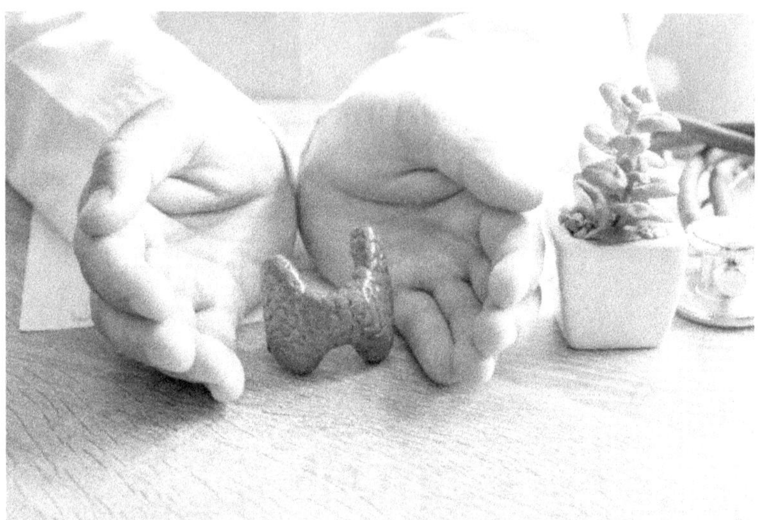

**Jack: Thyroid gland**: A gland that produces and stores hormones that aid in the regulation of heart rate, blood pressure, body temperature, and the rate at which food is converted into energy. Every cell in the body is dependent on the thyroid hormones that are present.

Thyroxine (T4) and triiodothyronine (T3) are the two most important thyroid hormones.

**Daniel**-What are the thyroid diseases?

**Jack**-The thyroid gland is linked to the following diseases:

Hyperthyroidism is characterised by an excess of hormones produced by the thyroid gland, which is in the front of the neck.

**Hyperthyroidism Symptoms**

- A fast heartbeat
- Rapid weight loss
- Tremors
- Sleeplessness
- Inconsistent Menstrual cycle

*Hypothyroidism* - A condition resulting from decreased production of thyroid hormones. Symptoms of Hypothyroidism vary between individuals, and they tend to develop slowly.

**Commonly noted symptoms include:**

- Fatigue

- Weight gain

- Increased blood cholesterol level

- Increased sensitivity to cold

- Constipation

- Dry skin

- Puffy face

- Hoarseness

- Muscle weakness, aches, tenderness, and stiffness

- Joint pain, stiffness, or swelling

- Irregular menstrual periods or amenorrhea

- Dry hair or hair loss

**Hypothyroidism in children could lead to:**

- Delayed and poor growth

- Delayed puberty

- Poor mental development

- Reasons for Thyroid

- Sedentary lifestyle

- Overuse of medicines

**Diet**

We must understand that, according to Naturopathy philosophy, the cause of any disease is the presence of foreign matter in the body, which can cause any disease. Foreign matter in the body interferes with the normal functioning of any organ, resulting in disease.

Our body is the best Thyroid specialist; however, only few people are aware of this.

The two primary functions of the body's vital energy are digestion and healing. However, we rarely allow our bodies to heal because we eat constantly throughout the day, beginning with a heavy breakfast, followed by lunch and dinner, at least twice a day tea or coffee, and snacking in between with packaged food, how can we expect our bodies to heal if we keep them busy with digestion all day? So, in the following topics, we will learn how to train our bodies to perform as doctors.

**Treatment of Thyroid-**

In the management of Thyroid following are the major pillars:

1. Diet

2. Intermittent fasting

3. Body Detoxification

4. Exercise

5. Sunlight

We will understand each pillar

**1. Diet:** In today's world, we have adopted many unhealthy food items that are not only bad for our bodies but also bad for our monthly budget. We need to get closer to natural foods, which will keep us healthy while also saving us money.

**Healthy Diet Plan**

Detox Juice -8 a.m.

As previously discussed, according to Naturopathy, the presence of toxins in the body is the primary cause of Thyroid issues, so our priority should be to eliminate toxins as soon as possible.

On an empty stomach, one glass of Ash Gourd (*Safed Petha*) juice works as a body cleanser. It quickly detoxifies the body. Before making juice, you peel it off and remove the seeds.

It is a natural substance that has no negative side effects.

Nothing should be consumed for at least thirty minutes after consuming the ash gourd juice, as this will interfere with the detoxification process.

**Breakfast**-10 a.m.

Only eat fresh fruits in the morning to stay nourished and energetic throughout the day.

Seasonal fruits should be preferred because there is an importance to having seasonal fruits that our mother nature has designed to meet the seasonal needs of the body.

Preferably, one type of fruit should be consumed daily, but you can mix and match the fruits based on your preferences and availability.

Tea and coffee should be avoided, but if you can't resist, take them after 60 minutes of finishing fruits.

**Lunch-1p.m.**

Lunch will be served on two plates, 50% salads and 50% freshly cooked food.

Plate one (carrot, onion, tomato, cucumber, beat root, radish, etc.)

Salads are eaten to provide enough fibre, minerals, vitamins, and water to aid in the detoxification of the body. Aside from that, we get the necessary nutrients.

Plate two: This plate should include fresh home-cooked food, such as chapati, green vegetables, dal, and so on.

**Dinner**-6p.m.

Dinner will be served the same as lunch, which will consist of two plates.

**Preferred food**

- Have coconut water instead of cold drinks.

- Have fresh coconut milk instead of animal milk.

**Prohibited food**

- Meat, fish, eggs, milk and milk products, paneer, ghee, cheese, and other animal-supplied foods should be avoided.

- All dead/packaged food should not be consumed as this kind of processed food makes us ill and doesn't provide any nutrients.

- We should avoid packaged juice and carbonated drinks.

- We should avoid Maida.

## 2. Intermittent fasting

We previously discussed how, to stay healthy, we should allow our bodies to heal themselves naturally, and that they should perform both the tasks of digestion and healing in a balanced manner. The idea behind intermittent fasting is that we should leave at least a 14–16-hour gap between dinner and the next day's breakfast so that our bodies can detoxify naturally.

If you look at the time between dinner and breakfast, you will notice that it is 16 hours, which will result in immediate healing results.

*Please refer to chapter one on fasting.*

## 3. Body detoxification

If we want to be healthy, we must keep our bodies clean on the inside, which has been emphasised repeatedly in the Naturopathic treatment of any disease.

An enema is an excellent way to cleanse the large intestine, which aids in the elimination of most diseases. It is a simple yet effective cleaning method that has been used since ancient times.

Enema Method: Fill an enema pot with 250ml of lukewarm water, which can be purchased at any nearby chemist shop. Apply coconut or mustard oil to the tip of the enema pot pipe and the anus to make it easier to insert the enema pot pipe into the anus. If you can, try to hold water inside for ten minutes. You'll only be able to hold it for a few minutes at first, but with practice, you'll be able to hold it for up to ten minutes. This process will detoxify your body thoroughly while causing no side effects. For further details, please refer to the full chapter on Enema.

Enema should be taken for 21 days at first, then once a week after that.

## 4. Exercise

We need to exercise to stay healthy. We should incorporate exercise into our daily routine. Any type of exercise, such as *running, yoga, cycling, zumba, brisk walking, or dancing,* is beneficial.

Daily minimum: 30 minutes. Please try to sweat while exercising; otherwise, the purpose will be defeated.

*Sarvangasna* (shoulder stand) is very effective in thyroid diseases because it improves blood flow to the neck region and thus quickly corrects thyroid diseases.

## 5.Sunlight

We spend a lot of time indoors, depriving our bodies of a great source of natural energy, sunlight. It not only gives us vitamin D but also keeps our bodies healthy. Toxins are killed by the warming effect. It is recommended that we spend 10-15 minutes in the sun to have a greater impact on our bodies.

**Time**: The best times to bask are one hour after sunrise and one hour before sunset. At that time, the therapeutic benefits are enormous without the risk of sunburn.

**Duration:** 15 minutes per day at the suggested time.

## Q&A

Q1: What if someone has been taking medication for a long time?

A-Medicines should not be stopped, but by adhering to the above plan, the need for the medications will be avoided, and the doctor will discontinue the medications.

Q2-How long will it take to eradicate this disease?

A-In most cases, patients experience relief within 21 days, but a complete cure may take 3–4 months.

Q3-Can I take outside food

A: It should be avoided for the first three months to achieve faster relief. Later, once every two weeks, a cheat day can be observed.

Q4- It is recommended that you avoid milk. How will I meet my calcium requirements?

A- Calcium is not only found in A-Milk. Nature has provided abundant calcium sources, and the following are excellent calcium sources that can be included in our diet:

- Coconut water
- Sesame (one spoon full of sesame seed will offer a significant amount of calcium)
- Fruits are the good source of calcium
- Coconut also provides calcium

# Chapter Ten

# HIGH BLOOD PRESSURE-A SILENT KILLER

- ➢ Definition
- ➢ Symptoms
- ➢ Treatment

# High Blood Pressure-A Silent Killer

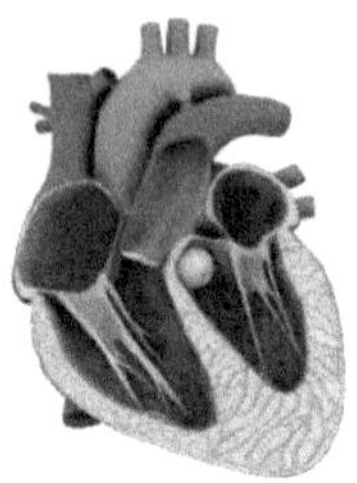

**Jack**- Our hearts, as we are all aware, supply blood to every part of the body. The heart must exert some pressure to pump the blood, which is normal. However, when the blood thickens, the heart must exert greater pressure to pump the blood throughout the body, which is known as hypertension or high blood pressure. When the systolic Blood Pressure readings on two different occasions are equal or above 140 mm hg and/or the diastolic Blood Pressure readings on both days are equal or above 90 mm hg, hypertension is diagnosed.

According to WHO estimates, there are 1.13 billion hypertensive people worldwide, with the majority (two-thirds) living in low- and middle-income countries.

High Blood Pressure (BP) is one of the most serious health issues confronting India today. According to the Journal of Hypertension's 2014 report on India, the overall hypertension prevalence is 29.8 percent, implying that 378.5 million Indian adults are hypertensive.

**Daniel**-Is there a sigh of relief after so much bad news?

**Jack**-Don't worry, among all the bad news, there is some good news. You can get rid of this deadly disease by changing your lifestyle and adopting healthy eating habits, and you can do so in as little as 3-4 months. Yes, friends, you read that correctly. High blood pressure can be reversed in as little as three months.

## High Blood Pressure Management

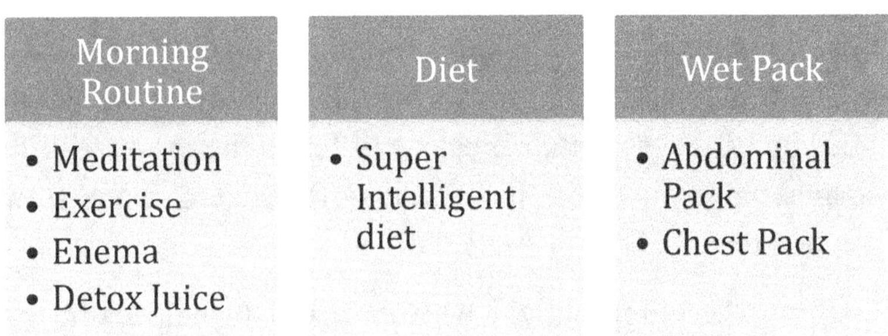



We have seen the three steps of the high blood pressure control programme mentioned above. Now we will understand this.

## 1. Morning Routine

**A Meditation**-morning routine can help to control high blood pressure levels. Because stress is the leading cause of high blood pressure, it is recommended that you meditate for at least an hour every day. This will significantly calm your mind, reducing stress levels to a large extent. It will be difficult at first to meditate for 30 minutes. You can start small and work your way up. You can begin with 2 minutes of meditation and gradually increase the duration of meditation, and the results will be amazing when you meditate. Don't forget to feed your mind daily with meditation. It will also boost your productivity.

**Exercise:** It is more important to burn calories than to consume them. It has been proven time and again that exercise is critical to our health. We rarely move our bodies in this day and age of digitalization and automation. With the click of a button, everything is at your fingertips. As a result, moving your muscles becomes even more important. You can do any exercise you want, such as badminton, cricket, running, jogging, brisk walking, or any other activity that raises your heart rate. The minimum duration for blood pressure patients is 30 minutes per day, but don't overstretch your body. Take regular breaks and finish the exercise with Shavasana to maximise the benefits of the exercise and slow the heartbeat.

Balloon Breathing should be done daily to help calm the patient and improve the body's functioning (please refer to chapter 2 for full details of Balloon Breathing).

**Enema**: Should be done consistently for three weeks, then reduced to once a week. Please see Enema Chapter 3 for more information.

**Detox Juice**: The faster the detoxification, the faster the relief. After having the process of enema with a gap of 30 minutes, the first thing to do is have a juice of ash gourd. It has wonderful detoxification properties; it clears the intestine pathway faster. This juice is to be consumed daily as it doesn't have any side effects. If you don't get ash gourd, you can have coconut water, which is called natural nectar (please read the detailed topic in previous chapters), or the juice of any vegetable will work.

**2. Smart Diet**-Please stick to the smart diet plan if you want to get rid of any acute or chronic disease. You will achieve incredible results. (Please refer to Chapter Six, "Super Intelligent Diet Regime," for more information.)

- **Say No to 3White poison: white** sugar, white salt, and maida are all poisonous. If you want to live a healthy life, eliminate this dangerous substance from your diet right away because it is not natural. They have been refined in the factory and thus have a negative impact on our bodies. Instead, you can substitute natural substances.

| Say No to | Say Yes |
| --- | --- |
| Sugar | Jaggery, Rock Sugar (mishri) |
| White salt | Rock salt |
| Maida | Wheat floor |

By replacing these whites, the process of healing will be much faster.

**3. Wet Pack-**Since ancient times, wet packs have been used to treat a variety of diseases. We can break the habit of occasionally taking poisonous medicines.

Method: Take a large cotton cloth large enough to cover your stomach. Wet the cloth and wrap it around your stomach so that the belly button is in the centre of the cloth. This improves blood circulation, which aids in the removal and elimination of toxins from the body.

 In the winter, wet packs should be avoided.

With all three steps of high Blood Pressure management, you will be able to eliminate the dreadful disease of high blood pressure and avoid heart attacks, myocardial infarction, strokes, and angioplasty.

# CHAPTER ELEVEN

# HYPERACIDITY

- ➤ Definition
- ➤ Symptoms
- ➤ Treatment

# Hyperacidity

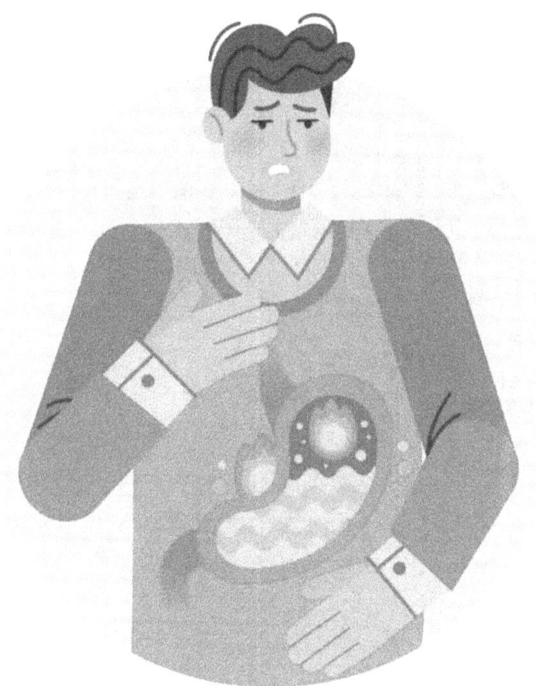

**Denial:** Finally, the CEO of the corporation threw an office party to celebrate the achievement of the month's revenue targets. It was a late-night affair, with food served around 11:30 p.m. I was not in the mood to walk after returning from the party because it was getting late, so I avoided it, but now I have a burning sensation in my chest and stomach. Please advise on a way out.

**Jack-** This is an indication of hyperacidity. Don't worry, we'll take care of it with natural ingredients.

**Defination**-Hydrochloric acid is produced in the stomach and is essential in the digestion process. It also kills bacteria found in food, protecting us from the risk of bacterial and fungal infections caused by contaminated food.

Hyperacidity refers to the body's excessive production of *HCL*. In everyday language, we refer to this as "acidity."

**Symptoms**

Hyperacidity can be painful and has several severe symptoms, which are listed below.

- Heart Burn

- Loss of appetite

- Flatulence

- Feelings of fullness

- In cases of GERD (acid reflux disease), hyperacidity can cause throat infections.

- If hyperacidity remains for a longer time, it will cause gastric ulcers.

- Hyperacidity can cause ulcerative colitis.

- If the body remains acidic for a longer period, it can cause cancer as well.

- Hyperacidity can damage food pipes.

In light of the foregoing symptoms, acidity should be treated in order to reduce the occurrence of chronic diseases.

**Treatment**

Fasting is the best way to treat hyperacidity (refer to the fasting chapter), but the following home remedies are recommended for immediate relief.

1. Collect **30 ml** of mint juice for home extraction. Add one spoon of lemon juice and 30 ml of water. Take this solution on an empty stomach early in the morning for seven days. It will not only relieve acidity but also improve the intestinal flora, which will improve digestion.
2. For instant relief from acidity, take one spoon of baking soda and mix it well in a glass of normal temperature water. You will feel good after taking this solution.
3. Place a spoonful of baked cumin seeds on a plate and set aside for a few minutes. Swallowing the baked seeds with a glass of water will give you instant relief.
4. Chewing clove buds after each meal, followed by a glass of lukewarm water, aids digestion.
5. In a food processor, combine a cup of crushed banana mix, two units of cardamom, and two spoons of rock sugar (*Mishri*) for a few seconds. Your acidity treatment is complete. If possible, take this mixture on an empty stomach; otherwise, it can be taken at any time.
6. Buttermilk can reduce the acidic effect. Fresh buttermilk can be consumed twice a day, or it can be fed in place of cooked food, which will provide powerful acidity results.
7. Applying a wet pack to the abdomen daily will eliminate toxins from the body, nourish the digestive system, and cause the toxins to become loose, allowing them to be

expelled quickly. (For more information on wet packs, see chapter four on wet packs.)

8. The patient with hyperacidity should consume only watermelon for breakfast, which will render greater relief immediately, and the regime of Super Intelligent Diet should be followed.

# CHAPTER TWELVE

## FEVER/FLU/COMMON COLD

- ➤ Introduction
- ➤ Treatment

# Fever/Flu/Common Cold

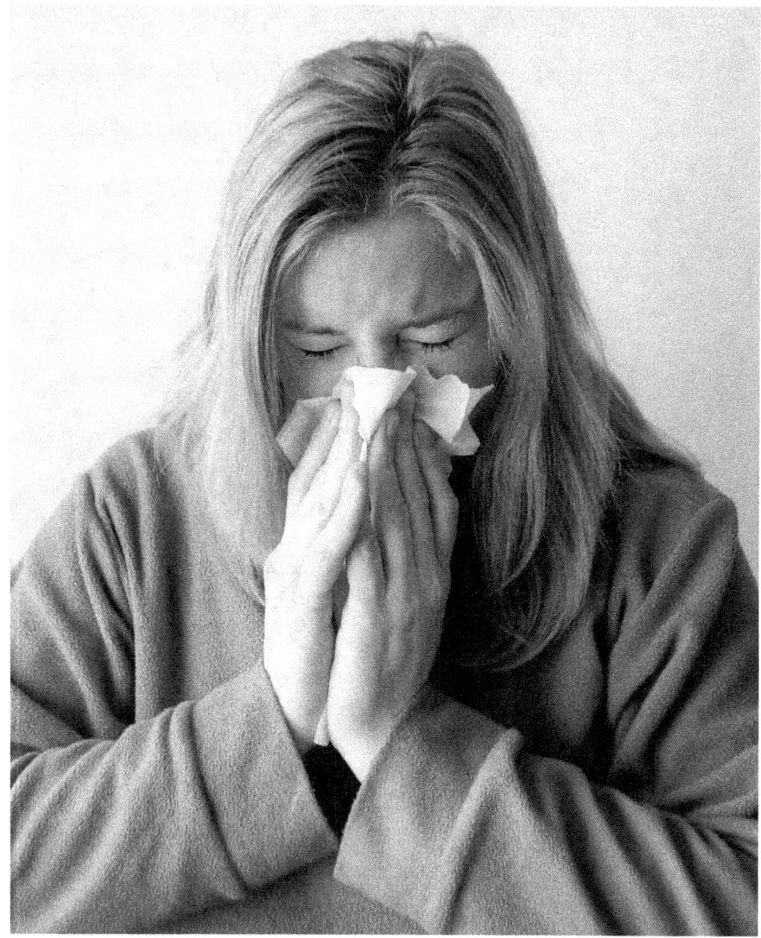

It's late at night, around 12 a.m. Jack was sound asleep when his phone rang. It took a while for him to notice the loud noise of the phone; he picked it up, and it was Daniel on the other end of the line; he sounded concerned because his son was running a fever. Jack's words made him feel a little better and guided him on how to get rid of the fever naturally.

**Jack**: As we all know, fever is one of the friendliest diseases, so don't worry. Instead, we should help our immune system improve its ability to fight foreign invaders. It is an indication of a battle between the body's immune system and the toxins present in the body. We must be cautious not to take any fever-reducing medication.

Hippocrates, the father of medicine, once said, ***"Give me fever, and I will cure everything."***

As previously stated, our bodies are intelligent enough to fight and cure all diseases on their own, and symptoms such as fever, cold, and cough indicate that the body's immune system is doing its job of cleaning toxins from the body. However, in today's modern world, everything that is quick and easy is quickly adopted, so we take allopathic medicines and suppress these mild and friendly symptoms at the expense of developing more severe diseases in the future. We simply need to encourage our bodies to adopt a healthy lifestyle, which will aid in the elimination of toxins and keep us healthy.

According to *Dr Lindlahr,* "Every so-called acute (Fever, Cold etc.) diseases result from cleaning and healing efforts of nature."

**Diet during Fever**

- Cooked foods should be avoided while suffering from a fever.

- Consumption of fruits and juices is recommended.

- Consume lemon water with honey.

- Every hour, we should drink water. It will aid in the elimination of toxins from the body through urine and sweat.

- Once the fever has subsided, a light diet of Dalia, Khichdi, and Sprouted grains should be consumed.

**Treatment 1:** Boil a cup of any black cold drink with two spoons of Ginger juice until it is reduced to half. Consume this delectable concoction twice a day. You will see miraculous results, and it can also be given to children.

**Treatment 2:** If a fever develops, skip meals, and instead drink citrus, fresh fruit juice, and coconut water throughout the day.

Method of Consuming Fresh Juices and Coconut Water: Start your day with coconut water and take any citrus juice (orange, lime, pineapple, etc.) at an interval of every two hours. The goal is to boost Vitamin C levels to boost immunity.

Quantity -If your weight is 70 Kg, consume 7 glasses of fresh citrus juice and 7 glasses of coconut water during the entire day.

Make certain that the juices and coconut water are fresh and natural. Nothing else should be consumed besides these two drinks, and no packaged drinks should be consumed. This process will greatly detoxify your body, and the fever should be gone in a couple of days. This procedure should be repeated the following day for half a day. On day two and three, you can consume light cooked foods, as well as coconut water and fruit juices.

**Treatment 3:** Roast one spoonful of carom seeds for a few seconds. Roast one spoon of rock salt until it turns a darkish pink. Combine both ingredients in a cup of hot water and sip this mixture. This is an excellent fever reliever.

**Treatment 4:** Wrap three to four ice cubes in a napkin before applying to the neck. Keep it on your skin until you're numb. Repeat the procedure until the temperature is reduced. This is a tried-and-true method for providing immediate relief from any type of fever.

**Treatment 5:** Clove has antibacterial and antiviral properties, making it useful in the treatment of a variety of diseases. Apply two drops of clove essential oil to your feet after mixing it with a carrier oil such as coconut, mustard, sesame, or almond oil. The results will astound you.

**Treatment 6:** A spoonful of onion juice mixed with a spoonful of honey, to be consumed 3–4 times per day depending on the severity of the fever. This is a method of lowering the temperature that does not involve the use of medication, and by doing so, we are assisting our bodies in naturally eliminating all toxins.

A wet bandage can be very useful in controlling high temperatures. Wet a cotton cloth in cold water, squeeze it, and wrap it around your head. It will not only reduce fever but will also relieve headache. (For more information on the use of wet bandages, please see the full chapter four on this subject.)

# Common Cold

It is, as the name implies, a very common symptom. This is not a disease; it is a symptom that our bodies are detoxifying and fighting diseases. As a result, it is a friendly disease that should not be suppressed with heavy and toxic medicines, which will turn it into a chronic disease.

The symptoms of a common cold

- Runny nose • Blocked nose • Breathing difficulties • Body heaviness • Lethargy • Chest congestion • Throat infections

**Reasons**

- Breathing polluted air
- Sleeping in a closed room with no air passage
- Overeating
- Indigestion
- Constipation
- Allergy due to strong fragrance
- Frequent consumption of fast food
- Presence of toxins (allergens) in the body.

**Therapy**

- ✓ Drink plenty of warm water.
- ✓ Enema should be administered with warm water.
- ✓ Consume the juices of spinach, turnip, carrot, tomato, ginger, and coriander. Sweating will cleanse the digestive system because of this juice. Every three hours, this juice should be consumed.

✓ The room's windows should be open, and fresh air should circulate throughout the night.

✓ Soaking your feet in warm water at night will provide immediate relief from your symptoms.

✓ *Jalneti* is effective in treating common cold symptoms, including a blocked nose.

✓ To get immediate relief from a blocked nose, sleep on the opposite side of the blocked nostril. For example, if the left nostril is blocked, one should lie down on the right side.

✓ To get rid of a runny and blocked nose, put two drops of mustard oil in each nostril three times a day.

✓ An intermittent fast should be observed daily to help clean the system faster.

## Precautions

- All dairy products, including ghee, curd, paneer, cheese, and milk, should be avoided during the illness.

- Toxic medicines should not be used because they can worsen the disease and lead to other fatal diseases.

# CHAPTER THIRTEEN

# ERECTILE DYSFUNCTION (ED)

- ➢ Introduction and Rationale
- ➢ Natural Treatment Method

# Erectile Dysfunction (ED)

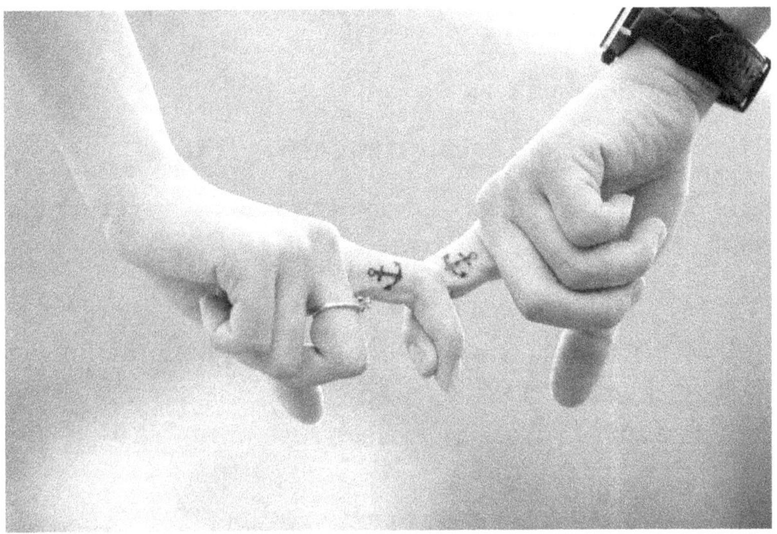

**Daniel**- Today, I'd like to learn more about a subject on which I'm a little hesitant to speak.

**Jack**- Please tell me about your concern; don't be shy; as your mentor, I should be aware of everything concerning you and your health.

**Daniel:** I am unable to enjoy my sexual life because I am unable to perform at my peak level.

**Jack**-ED is very common today and can wreak havoc on human relationships. The major causes of ED are said to be higher stress levels in young people, sedentary lifestyles, excessive use of digital devices, and foods rich in fat and spices.

Today, we are disconnected from nature and live an artificial life, which increases the likelihood of new modern-age diseases. Most young children's daily routines have been drastically altered, which means they are awake all night and sleep in the morning hours, which is harmful to the human body. Adding a slew of complications that will become apparent later in life.

**The Definition of Erectile Dysfunction (ED)**

ED is defined as a lack of desire or capability to perform in bed.

As a result, it has been discovered that the primary cause of ED is a lack of blood circulation to the genitals, resulting in a lack of genital erection, and the secondary cause is stress, which results in a lack of desire to perform.

Anything good for your heart is said to be good for your genitals. The rationale for this is poor blood circulation, which is hampered by either cholesterol or stress. Both situations are harmful to one's heart and sexual life. As a result, the first step toward a healthy sexual life is to maintain a healthy diet and routine.

Meditation plays an important role in controlling the flow of excessive thoughts, thereby significantly lowering stress levels.

ED can be successfully treated with a change in lifestyle and the suggestions listed below:

**Treatment 1**: Because we know that the primary cause of ED is a lack of blood circulation, our goal is to detoxify our bodies so that toxins are eliminated, and blood circulation is improved.

The best way to detoxify is to fast on a regular basis, which will not only detoxify your body but also increase your vitality, and you will be able to permanently eliminate this disease.

**Treatment 2:** Sesame oil is a great choice for increasing muscle strength and blood circulation. Regularly massage your genitals and surrounding areas with sesame oil to improve blood circulation and reduce the occurrences of ED.

**Treatment 3**: Nature has been extremely generous to humans. It has provided us with a highly effective natural substance known as *Shilajit*. This is an excellent supplement for both types of ED, namely lack of desire and inability to perform. This supplement provides a comprehensive approach to addressing the ED problem. *Shilajit* not only strengthens your muscles but also significantly calms your mind, making this wonder supplement a holistic cure. *Shilajit* is available in a variety of forms on the market, including tablets, capsules, powder, and raisin forms. We should only take Shilajit in raisin form to reap the most benefits, as nature has only provided it in this form; the other forms have been altered.

**Dosage**: A pea-sized amount should be mixed with any hot beverage, such as milk, coffee, or water, and taken after breakfast or at bedtime. It is recommended to take it twice in the winter and once in the summer.

## Meditation's Influence

Because of modern lifestyle, corporate work pressure, higher financial ambitions, and other factors, stress has been a major contributor to erectile dysfunction in today's youth. To get rid of stress, which is a major cause of many lifestyle diseases, it is critical to control stress levels and begin living a happy life. Meditation is the most effective way to control your thoughts, which significantly reduces stress levels. It will not only get you out of this danger, but it will also keep you fresh and energetic throughout the day.

Meditation will change you in every aspect of your life. I understand how difficult it is to meditate on your own. You can work with a coach or mentor to help you achieve this goal. Some of the suggested meditation techniques are listed below.

- Brahma Kumari's Meditation
- Meditation by Sadguru
- Vipassana by DhammaThali
- Meditation by Sri Sri

Exercise on a daily basis-ED is caused by a lack of blood circulation to the genital area, so our goal should be to increase blood circulation. Exercise is the most effective way to increase blood flow.

**Suggested Exercises**

- Morning/Evening Walk
- Brisk Walk
- Yoga is the best way to keep your body and mind agile
- Zumba and dancing are also great ways to exercise and boost your mood

Tip-Start with five minutes daily, your mind will not resist you staying away, it is a good habit-forming tip after that you can gradually increase time until you make it a routine.

# CHAPTER FOURTEEN

## A GOOD NIGHT'S SLEEP

- ➤ Definition
- ➤ Solution

# A Good Night's Sleep

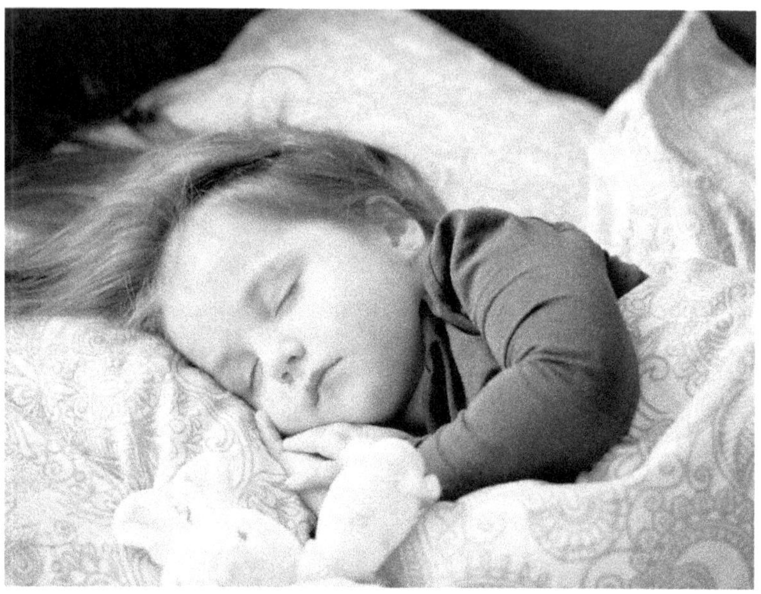

It was a bright and sunny morning. Jack and Daniel were strolling through the lush, green garden. Jack took off his shoes and began walking. Daniel was whining about his lack of sleep.

Dr. Jack stepped in and, with his wisdom, briefed everyone on the importance of good sleep.

As our phones must be charged daily to function properly throughout the day, our bodies must be charged through sound sleep in order to function properly.

Sleep is a natural occurrence that occurs for 7-8 hours every night, during which the nervous system is relatively inactive, the eyes are closed, the muscles are relaxed, and consciousness is nearly suspended. Deep, or restorative, sleep is as essential to health as oxygen or food.

The following are the benefits of sound or deep sleep.

- Short sleep causes obesity or weight gain.

- The person who sleeps well eats less.

- It improves concentration and memory.

- Deep sleep enhances physical performance.

- Deep sleep reduces the risk of heart disease and stroke.

- Deep sleep increases glucose metabolism and reduces the risk of diabetes.

- Deep sleep reduces the risk of depression.

- Eight hours of deep sleep can improve your immune system.

- Deep sleep improves the digestive system.

- Deep sleep improves your emotional quotient.

**Reasons for less sleep**

- Mental or physical workload

- Stress is the biggest reason for insomnia.

- Smoking

- Drugs and alcohol

- Having food late at night

- Sleeping in a non-ventilated room

- Inadequate physical activity.

- Taking medicines makes the nervous system weak and causes insomnia.

- Sleeping in noisy surroundings

**What is the challenge?**

The faster world of today has given us less sleep due to many factors such as stress, fast life, less time due to a lot of accomplishment pressure, and spending more time on screens, especially on mobile devices at night, which causes less sleep and that is not sound sleep, but don't worry, there is a solution for every problem.

**Managing sleep effectively means**

- Take a shower before going to bed. Showering relaxes not only your body but also your mind, promoting sound sleep. I know it's difficult in the winter, but you can energise yourself with lukewarm water.

- Lavender essential oil is the most effective way to relax your mind. Apply 3-4 drops of essential oil to your pillow and you will immediately fall asleep. You can use an essential oil diffuser to create a sleep-inducing environment in your bedroom.

- *Anulom Vilom* should be done right before going to bed. It will not only improve the oxygen supply to brain cells, but it will also significantly calm your mind and make you want to sleep immediately.

- If done right before bed, soaking your feet in lukewarm water mixed with table salt promotes deep sleep.

- Massage lukewarm mustard oil into your feet and head to relax the muscles and promote restful sleep.

- Deep breathing exercises should be done before going to bed to reduce thoughts and calm your mind.

- At bedtime, two drops of *ANU TAIL* in the nostrils relax brain cells and promote deep sleep.

- At bedtime, two drops of pure cow ghee inserted in the nostril will improve sleep quality.

- A gentle scalp massage with oil mixed with two drops of lavender oil will help you sleep better.

- Exercise, yoga, and a brisk walk in the morning and evening will improve blood circulation and thus promote sound sleep.

- Please dress comfortably before going to bed. Clothes should not be too tight because they will obstruct blood circulation and cause discomfort.

- Finally, turn off all digital friends at least an hour before going to bed, which means keeping your lifeline (cell phone) away from your bed.

*Anu Tail is an ayurvedic proprietary medicine that can be purchased at any ayurvedic store near you. The leading manufacturers are Dabur and Patanjali.*

# Chapter Fifteen

## EAR NOSE & THROAT

- ➢ Sinusitis
- ➢ Nasal Polyps
- ➢ Running Nose
- ➢ Blocked Nose
- ➢ Asthma
- ➢ Cough

# Ear Nose & Throat

Sinusitis /Nasal Polyps/Allergic Rhinitis

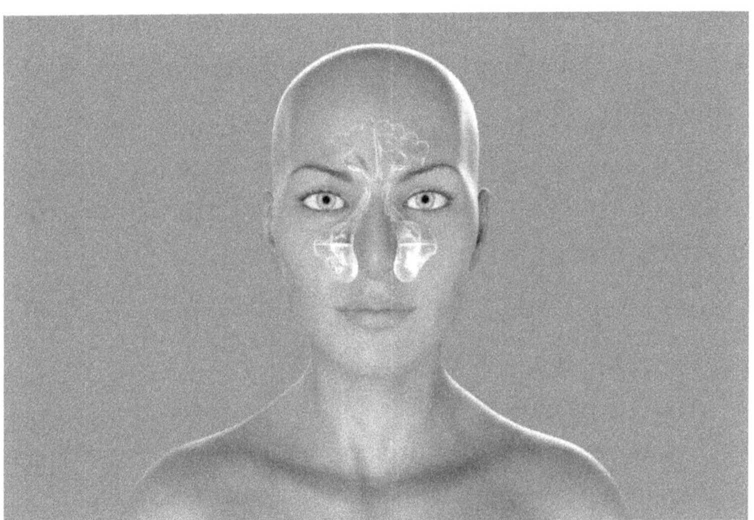

**Jack-** The rapid growth of industrialization has raised the *per capita income,* which has resulted in increased purchasing power and the pursuit of items of luxury, which in turn has scaled up the number of vehicles on the road. Consequently, pollution in the environment has increased, causing several respiratory disorders in humans. Today, as per a study conducted by the *Indian Medical Association,* every seventh person suffers from breathing disorders like sinusitis, asthma, running nose, and allergic rhinitis. This can wreak havoc in the future.

**Daniel-** Is it true? If so, what could be the possible solution to it?

**Jack-** Don't worry! There is a solution for every problem in nature; we will learn to resolve ENT disorder with the help of nature's cure.

*Sinusitis* is an inflammation or swelling of the tissue lining the sinuses. *Sinuses* are hollow spaces within the bones between your eyes, behind your cheekbones, and in your forehead. They make mucus, which keeps the inside of your nose moist. That helps protect against dust, allergens, and pollutants.

Healthy sinuses are filled with air. But when they become blocked and filled with fluid, germs can grow and cause an infection.

**Causes of Sinusitis**

- The common cold
- Allergic rhinitis
- Small growths in the nose lining are called nasal polyps.
- Deviated septum, which is a shift in the nasal cavity

**Symptoms**

- Facial pain
- Stuffed nose
- Runny nose
- Cough and congestion.
- loss of smell.

**Remedies for Nasal Polyps, Sinusitis, and Nasal Blockage**

- Apply three drops of *ANU TAIL* thrice a day, which will clear the nasal passage, thus offering a substantial amount of relief from congestion and pain associated with it. Using *ANU TAIL* is to be prolonged, which will clear the sinusitis and other related diseases to a great extent.

- Steam is to be taken twice a day by mixing *Eucalyptus Essential Oil* (three drops). This will provide instant relief from nasal congestion and sinusitis-related symptoms.

- A weak immune system is the major cause of sinus-related ailments. A stronger immune system will aid in the fight against these diseases. The patient should consume 3 glasses of citric juice (orange, pineapple, or sweet lemon) daily, which will supply the desired amount of Vitamin C to boost the immune system.

- *Jalneti*-As per naturopathy treatment, *Jalneti* is an excellent practice to clear your nasal passage, thus providing dramatic relief in the symptoms of Sinusitis, Nasal polyps, Runny and stuffy nose.

- Lukewarm water mixed with common salt to be used for *Jalneti* can be performed regularly to not only cure the nasal disease but also to prevent these diseases in the future as well.

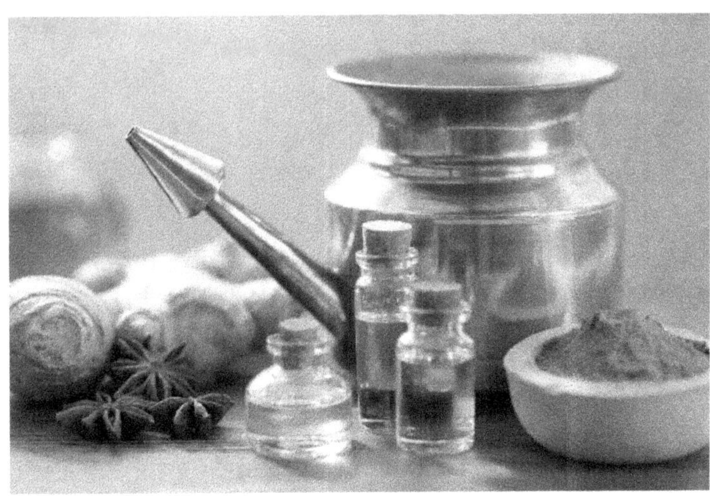

# Asthma

Lots of research has proved that the primary causes of asthma are mentioned below.

- Food allergy

- Allergies caused by pollution

- Dysfunction of the trachea

- Psychological disorders

- a result of the suppression of acute disease by medicine.

- Hence, keeping the above points in mind, we will discuss the therapy.

## Diet Recommendations

- The diet should be high in carbohydrates.

- should have sprouts in abundance.

- Fresh fruits are the keys to good health.

- Asthmatic patients should be an integral part of the diet of dry fruit.

- Salads and raw vegetables

- Goat's milk

- daily diet schedule.

- lemon juice in warm water.

- Milk and fruit

- Food: 50% salads, 50% food in each meal.

- Go for gooseberry juice three times a day in between meals.

- Intermittent fasting is super beneficial in controlling asthma.

**Therapy**

- A wet pack on the chest helps in clearing the toxins, clears the air passage and provides instant relief from asthmatic attacks.

- Exercise in the open air and balloon breathing is helpful.

- A complete steam bath in eucalyptus leaves is very helpful.

- Inhaling the steam from water with eucalyptus, essential oil, or leaves offers immediate relief.

- A warm foot bath twice a week should be performed.

A 2013 study published in the American Journal of Physiology showed quercetin found in onions can help relax airways and muscles, providing relief from asthma symptoms. It is evident from the above study that consumption of onions is quite useful in reducing the symptoms associated with asthma.

How to use: 1 spoon of onion juice to be mixed with raw honey and consumed on an empty stomach daily will relax the airways and reduce the attacks of asthma significantly.

- Insert three drops of *ANU TAIL* in both the nostrils. It will provide relief in symptoms associated with asthma with no side effects.

- *Jalneti*-As per naturopathy treatment, *Jalneti* is an excellent practice to clear your nasal passage, thus providing dramatic relief in the symptoms of Asthma.

With all the above steps, chronic and severe asthma can be cured

# Cough/Throat infections

As previously stated, cough is one of the friendliest types of symptoms.Cough is not a disease; it is a symptom that indicates the body is infected with some foreign matter, and it should not be suppressed with high doses of medicine; instead, we should aid our system in expelling the foreign matter from the body.Below are effective ways to support our body in expelling toxic materials:

- A higher intake of Vitamin C will help our body fight effectively against foreign materials. We should drink fresh fruit juices like pineapple, oranges, lime, etc. Vitamin C tablets should not be consumed.

- Fresh turmeric is the best antibiotic provided by nature. Grate fresh turmeric with the help of a grater. You will get a fresh juice out of it. Swallow that fresh turmeric juice and keep quiet for 15 minutes. A layer of turmeric will be formed in the throat which will help in eliminating the bacteria present in the throat, thus offering dramatic relief from any type of throat infection, cough, etc.

- Gargle with normal temperature water mixed with alum *(Fitkari)* powder. This will immediately lower the cough bouts and can be done more than a couple of times a day.

- Gargle with normal temperature water mixed with baking soda (one spoon). This will help in overcoming the throat and oral bacterial infections, thus providing immediate relief from cough and throat irritation.

- Gargle with any of the mouthwashes available at home. Mouthwash is antibacterial and antifungal, just like the cough and throat infections, so mouthwash provides instant relief from cough and throat infections.
- Gargle with *Betadine* oral solution is also helpful in throat infections.
- Apply eucalyptus essential oil with coconut oil and rub gently on the chest, ribs, feet, and on the shoulder blades. This will reduce chest congestion and enhance breathing.

# Chapter Sixteen

# PILES

- ➢ Causes
- ➢ Treatment

# Piles

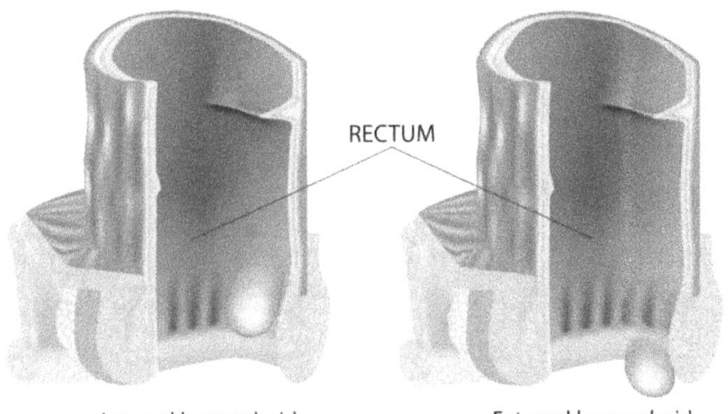



**Jack**-Piles is one of the most common diseases nowadays. It causes pain and irritation in the anus, and defecation becomes painful. Small and large lumps are formed in and around the anus, which can be felt upon touching. When these lumps enlarge, they form warts, and in contact with hard stool, they burst and cause bleeding.

**Daniel-** Are there different types of piles?

**Jack**: Yes, there are two types of piles.

External Piles: These are painful lumps on or around the orifice of the anus. They can cause pain on touching, but this causes little or no bleeding.

Internal Piles: Internal piles are formations inside the anus with a lot of blood loss. These make the patient look pale and aemic due to heavy blood loss.

**Causes of Piles**

- Sedentary lifestyle
- Constipation
- Consumption of alcohol.
- Consumption of oily and spicy foods
- Stress
- Dietary absence of fruits and salads
- Smoking
- Packaged food

**Management of Piles**: It is important to cure piles timely. Unattended piles for a longer time may increase the risk of cancer, so it is necessary to take immediate remedial steps by modifying our lifestyle and food habits.

Below are the main pillars of pile treatment.

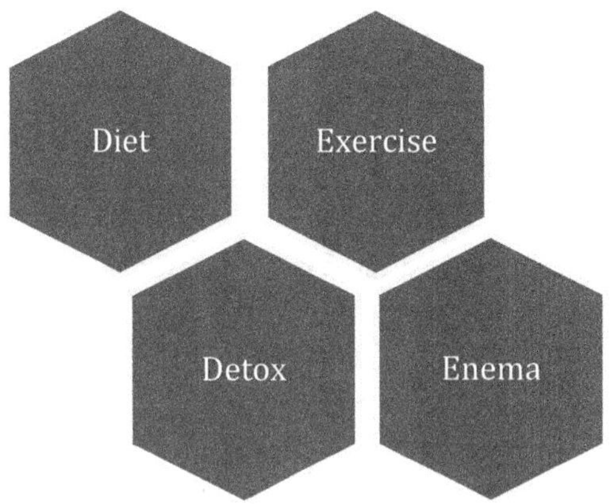



## 1. Diet

Diet plays a vital role in the management of piles as we need to avoid meat, fish, eggs, spicy and oily foods. We need to shift to a super intelligent diet and by adopting this diet regime, you will get rid of piles faster.

Please refer to chapter 6, "Super intelligent diet regime."

Consuming dry figs soaked in water overnight can be adequately beneficial for patients with piles. Take 3-4 units of dry figs, soak them in water for the night and have them in the morning with water.

## 2. Exercise

Exercise: Burning calories is extremely significant compared to getting them. It has been repeatedly proven that exercising is essential to keep you healthy. In the age of digitization and automation, our bodily movements have been reduced to almost zero as everything is just available on a click. Therefore, it is essential to flex our muscles. You can choose any exercise of your choice: playing badminton, cricket, running, jogging, brisk walking, or any other activity that accentuates your heartbeat. The minimum duration for piles patients is 45 min. daily, but don't overstretch your body to perform. Take regular breaks and end the exercise with *Shavasan*, which will help gain the maximum benefits of the exercise and slow down the heartbeat.

Practising *Uttanpaadasan, Pawanmuktasan, and Naukasan* will immensely benefit the patients' piles.

## 3. Enema

By now we are well versed with the concept that toxins are the main cause of any disease, which means they should be flushed out of the body quickly to get instant and prolonged relief.

You can buy Enema pot from any chemist, or you can buy it online as well.

The following steps should be followed for Enema:

- Apply coconut or mustard oil on the tip of the pipe of the pot and to the anus.

- Fill the pot with 300-400 ml of lukewarm water.

- Lie down on the mat, insert the pipe slowly into the anus.

- Water enters the stomach.

- Try to hold the water in your stomach for as long as you can, as it will remove toxins from the large intestine.

- Release the water as you feel to do so.

- Don't eat/Drink anything for at least 30 minutes, as the detoxification process is on. Initially, to be performed for 21 days, thereafter once in a week.

## 4. Detoxification

The faster the detoxification, the faster the relief. After having the process of enema, with a gap of 30 minutes, the first thing to do is have a juice of cucumber. It has a wonderful and amazing detoxification property; it clears the intestine pathway faster. This juice is to be consumed daily as it doesn't have any side effects.

Cucumber not only clears the intestines but also maintains the pH as well, which will soothe your digestive system immensely, and you will have relief from hyperacidity as well.

If you don't get cucumber, you can have coconut water, which is called natural nectar (please read the detailed topic in chapter 5), or the juice of any vegetable will work.

# CHAPTER SEVENTEEN

## MIGRAINE

- ➤ Definition
- ➤ Treatment

# Migraine

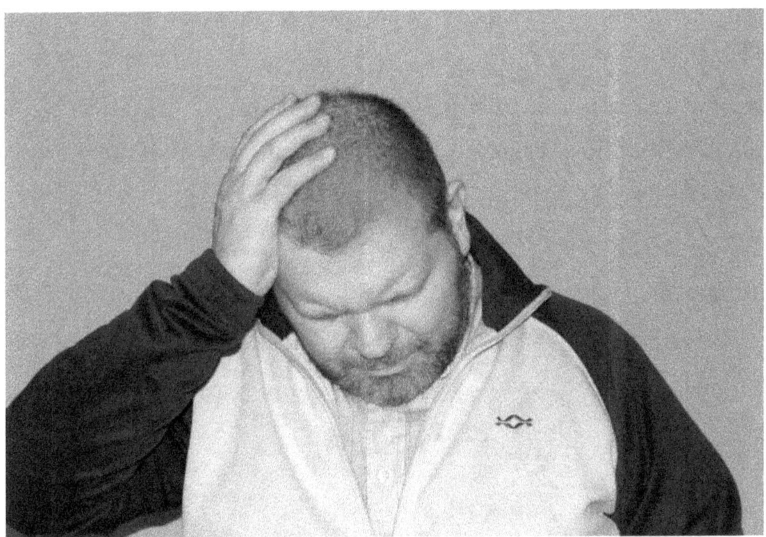

## Definition

**Jack-** Migraine is a headache that occurs on either the right or left side of the head. The pain is severe, the patient is irritated, and he can feel the pain even while sneezing or moving his head up and down.

**Danial**: Is there a consistent migraine pattern, Jack?

**Jack**: Migraine occurs at a specific time, which can be in the morning, evening, or at bedtime. In general, it happens because of any trigger, such as staring at a screen for long periods of time or because of the effect of a bright light bulb or welding.

## Symptoms

- Severe headache
- Nausea
- Vomiting

- Loss of appetite
- Tears
- Eye discomfort

There are two types of migraine. The first is migraine with aura, which is the rarest type of migraine in which the patient experiences a sparkling, rainbow-like light in either of the eyes. This aura lasts between 30 and 60 minutes.

The other type of migraine does not have an aura, but the rest of the symptoms are the same.

Migraine headaches can last up to seven days.

## Reasons

- Dryness of brain cells
- Sinusitis, nasal polyps, and other nasal disorders.
- Stress
- Side effects of medicine
- Smoking
- Consumption of alcohol.
- Weakness
- A shortage of sleep
- Lack of exercise

## Recommended diet

- A migraine patient should have a balanced diet. He should avoid excessive and spicy foods.

- should consume alkaline foods like fruits and vegetables.

- Sprouted grains should be consumed frequently.

- Fig, Gooseberry, Apple, Pomegranate, and Guava are excellent choices.

- Tea and coffee should be avoided.

- A non-vegetarian diet should be avoided.

- The food should have less salt and oil.

**Remedy**

- The patient should massage his or her head with pure cow ghee.
- Two times daily, insert three drops of pure cow ghee into both nostrils. It works wonders for migraines and greatly nourishes brain cells.
- Apply three drops of Anu Tail to both nostrils three times per day.It not only relieves migraines but also clears the airways.
- Jalneti is extremely beneficial for migraines.
- A wet bandage should be applied to the head and abdomen to ensure proper blood circulation and, as a result, migraine relief.
- Drinking water will provide immediate relief from a severe headache.
- One ancient migraine treatment is to drink jalebi with milk, which is said to provide instant energy to brain cells and thus provide excellent results.
- Meditation and yoga are simple choices that have a long-term impact.
- Soak your feet in warm water mixed with *EPSOM* salt, then apply a cold wet bandage to your forehead; you will notice an immediate improvement in your blood circulation and feel much more relaxed.

# Chapter Eighteen

# PIMPLES (ACNE)

- ➢ Causes
- ➢ Treatment

# Pimples (Acne)

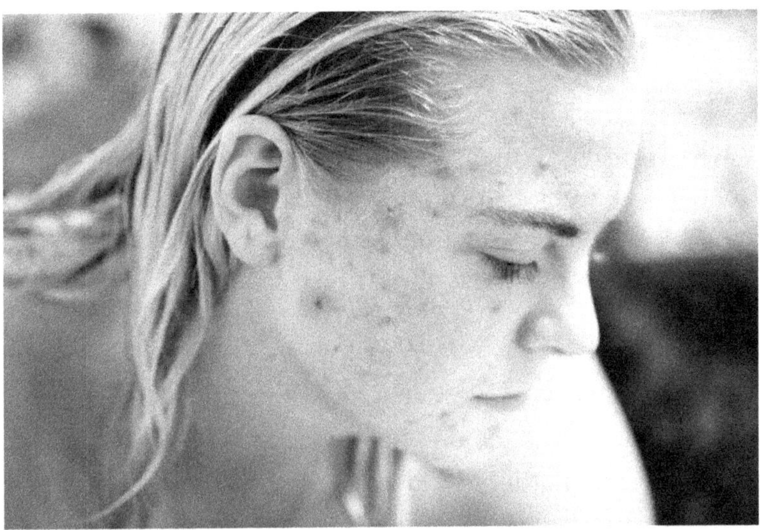

**Jack**-Acne is the most common disease in teenagers. It is because of the burning sensation of the glands in the pores of the skin. Acne develops on the face, neck, chest, and shoulders. It occurs between the ages of twelve and twenty-five years.

There are many types of acne, and all of them are related to the glands of hair follicles.

## Acne Factors

- As per the principles of naturopathy, the main cause of acne is toxic materials present in the body.
- Bad food habits cause acne.
- Sedentary lifestyles and lack of exercise aggravate the problem.
- Consumption of excessive fast food, which offers excessive starch, sugar, fat, and oil, makes the blood impure, thus causing acne.

- Constipation is a major cause of acne.

**Daniel**- There are numerous advanced creams on the market today that claim to provide instant relief from acne. Are those the best options?

**Jack-** No, they will exacerbate the problem because they contain a lot of toxic medicines, such as steroids, which have a lot of side effects, and the acne will reoccur. So, stick to natural treatments that will get to the root of the problem.

**Treatment**

- The patient should practise fasting for two days. He can have water and lemon juice only.
- After completing the fasting, he should consume fruits and fresh fruit juices only, which will enable the toxic material to come out of the body.
- Constipation should be eliminated with the help of enemas.
- A wet bandage to be applied to the abdomen regularly.
- The patient should take a steam of water mixed with tea tree oil for seven days, which will work as an antibacterial, thus providing a remedial effect.
- Multani (clay) mud paste to be applied on the area affected by acne, which will draw out all the local toxins present there.
- Ice works wonders to cure acne. Gently massage with a cube of ice the affected area. It will soothe your skin as well.
- Aloe Vera Gel is a wonderful remedy for acne. Apply fresh Aloe Vera gel on the affected area thrice a day.
- Apply tea tree essential oil with Aloe Vera gel. It will work like an antibiotic gel. to be applied twice daily.

- Wash your face with a banana peel with lemon juice twice daily, you will see a remarkable improvement.
- Aloe Vera gel mixed with lemon juice to be applied and kept overnight. It will have remedial impact on acne prone skin.
- *Please refrain from using any medication to treat acne. It will give you an immediate result, but it will also cause you extra problems in terms of side effects.*

# CHAPTER NINETEEN

# GALL BLADDER STONE

- ➢ Causes
- ➢ Symptoms
- ➢ Treatment

# Gall Bladder Stone

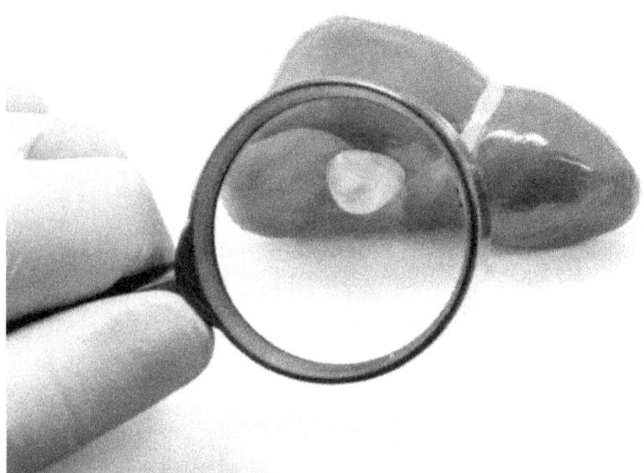

**Jack**-The main function of a gallbladder is to store bile, which is secreted by the liver. It is a pear-shaped organ and is attached to the liver on the right side. Bile is a composition of salts, acids, pigments, and cholesterol.

**Daniel**-What is bile used for?

Bile is useful for the digestion of fats.

**Gallstones Causes:**

The disturbance in the composition of bile changes the ratio of cholesterol and salts, which causes the formation of deposits. Initially, it is less in quantity, but with time, it increases in size, which leads to the formation of larger stones. The swelling in the gallbladder's lining may lead to the formation of particles.

The primary causes of the formation of gallstones are wrong food habits and a sedentary lifestyle, which makes the liver sick. Bile produced by the liver is of inferior quality, which causes the formation of stones.

**Symptoms**

- Mild pain and heaviness below the right rib area.
- Constipation
- Lack of appetite
- Jaundice
- A cold and fever
- After these mild symptoms, unbearable pain is felt.
- Sometimes the body shakes and there is cold sweat.
- Nausea and vomiting.

**Treatment**

- The patient should sit in a hot tub for 30 minutes.

- A cold bandage should be wrapped around the area below the ribs, above the naval, and should be covered with woollen cloth.

- A hot water bottle can also be placed under the rib area. The discomfort will pass.

- The patient should breathe deeply.

- Fasting will help immensely to get the stone out.

- Enema with hot water should be taken.

- A walk in the morning should not be avoided.

- Fresh fruits should be a part of your daily diet.

- Fresh fruit juice should be preferred.

- Buttermilk can be consumed.

- Watermelon is extremely beneficial.

**Should Be Avoided.**

- Ghee
- Milk
- Banana
- Dry fruits
- Fried food
- Potato

# CHAPTER TWENTY

## WEIGHT LOSS

- ➢ Reasons
- ➢ Treatment

# Weight loss

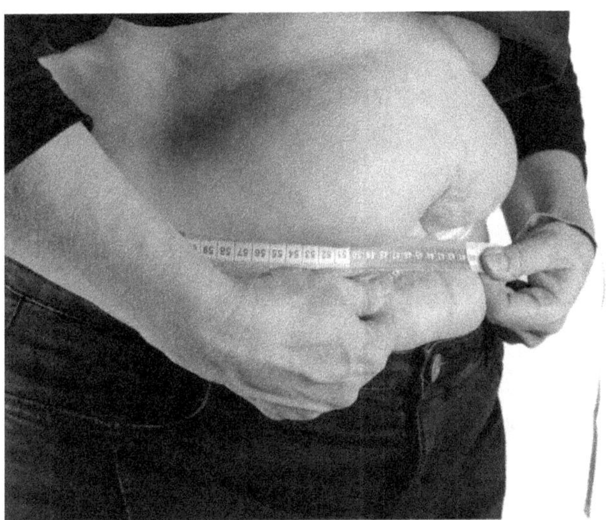

**Jack-**Obesity occurs when the body has an abnormally high level of fat deposition. Obesity is a disease that can lead to a variety of other diseases such as *heart disease, diabetes, varicose veins, constipation, skin disease, joint pain, arthritis, impotency, infertility,* and so on. Obesity can strike at any age or gender.

*Obesity=Calories intake > Calories Burnt*

**Daniel: According to what I've read, obesity** is a serious medical condition that puts additional strain on the legs, heart, lungs, kidneys, liver, and nervous system. This can shorten a person's life.

**Reasons**

- Unhealthy eating habits
- Sedentary lifestyle
- Lack of physical activity
- Sleeping more than necessary

- Weak digestive system
- Sleeping late at night
- Stress
- Consuming food more frequently.
- Intake of fast food

**Normal weight of kids**

| Age-Years | Boys (KG) | Girls (KG) |
|-----------|-----------|------------|
| 5 | 19.3 | 13.7 |
| 10 | 32.4 | 29.6 |
| 15 | 52.3 | 48.8 |
| 16 | 55.5 | 49.8 |

**Average weight of men and women according to height**

| Height-Feet | Men | Women |
|-------------|------|-------|
| 4.8 | 55 | 48 |
| 5.0 | 56.3 | 50.8 |
| 5.2 | 58.9 | 53.1 |
| 5.4 | 60.9 | 56.3 |
| 5.6 | 62.2 | 58.9 |
| 5.8 | 65.8 | 62.2 |
| 5.10 | 68.4 | 65.8 |
| 6.0 | 73 | 68.5 |

**Treatment:** The goal of the treatment is to get rid of the fat that has already accumulated in the body and to prevent it from accumulating further.

Fasting on water only for the first two days, if possible.

Fasting on orange juice for two days in a row reduces deposited fat at a faster rate.

After two days of fasting, one should consume orange juice, fresh fruits, and salads throughout the day. You can eat once a day (one chapati and one vegetable with salad). This regimen should be followed for at least 15 days. By then, you should have lost at least 5 kg. If you get hungry during the day, eat fruit instead of full meals.

In the morning, drink 4-5 glasses of warm water on an empty stomach.

Take an enema every day with either warm or cold water, depending on the weather.

Cucumber juice should be consumed daily.

Following significant weight loss, observe fasting once a week and adhere to the Super Intelligent Diet protocol (refer to the full guidelines in Chapter 6).

- A daily brisk walk is recommended.

- If at all possible, run

- A steam bath should be taken once a week to expel excess fat.

- Yoga and Zumba should also be included in the daily curriculum.

**Following Food should be avoided.**

- Ghee
- Rice
- Milk
- Oil
- Tea
- Coffee
- Meat

- Alcohol
- Sweets
- Chocolates
- Shakes
- Ice cream
- Flavored milk

*CAUTION:* *Do not take weight-loss medications or artificial juices because they can have dangerous side effects.*

# ANSWERS TO QUESTIONS

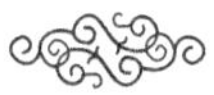

**Jack**-Daniel, congratulations on completing the entire module of nature's cure treatment for various diseases. I'm confident you'll make the most of it and spread the word about the benefits of this therapy.

There will be times when implementing these theories will be difficult, but you must be committed to it. You will try to take a shorter route to having medicine, which may be due to panic and time constraints, but you must be firm; naturopathy may take time, but it will be beneficial in the long run.

I've created a series of Q&As to help you clear your doubts.

**Question 1**: I've never used natural treatment methods before; will they work on me, as I'm usually dependent on allopathic medications?

**Answer**-Yes, they will help you get rid of any disease, even if you haven't received natural treatment, but keep in mind that it will take some time to cure because you've been using toxins medicines, but you will see results.

**Question 2**: Should I take any medications while I'm sick with a fever? What should you do if the temperature rises above 102 degrees Fahrenheit?

**Answer**-The medicine should be avoided completely; any fever can be brought down with the help of a wet bandage and other methods suggested.

**Question 3**: What if I'm on high blood sugar and high blood pressure medications?

**Answer**-Do not discontinue any medications; instead, continue with natural treatment; your blood pressure will drop dramatically, and your doctor will reduce the dose.

**Question 4**: Could you please advise on the proper way to take a bath?

**Answer**-In the winter, begin pouring water from the feet to the head; this will promote smooth blood circulation and reduce the risk of stroke and heart attack. In the summer, the opposite should be done.

**Question 5**: I have never fasted and have no plans to do so; please suggest an alternative solution.

**Answer** -If you are unable to fast for the entire day, please practice intermittent fasting, which is extremely beneficial and will yield the desired results; however, one full day of fasting is recommended first, followed by intermittent fasting.

**Question 6**-When is the best time to consume fruits?

**Answer** -First, we must understand how digestion works; fruits digest in about 30 minutes, so we should not eat them after a meal; instead, we can eat fruits first, then eat our meal, which will keep us away from acidity and bloating.

**Question 7**-Diabetic patients should avoid drinking coconut water and eating coconut fruits.

**Answer** -If you follow the standard diet plan and consume coconut water and fruits along with it, your blood sugar levels will rise; however, if you follow the intelligent diet suggested in the book, your blood sugar levels will remain stable.

**Question 8**-Will fasting cause me to become weak?

**Answer** -Fasting is a natural way to cleanse the body and should be done on a regular basis. Fasting does not make us weaker; rather, it strengthens our immune system. During fasting, our body's reserve fuel is used to provide energy, so don't worry, you won't feel weak.

**Question 9**-Is Naturopathy a scientifically proven therapy?

**Answer** -Naturopathy is the oldest form of medical system. It is referred to as the "mother of all systems." Fasting and treatment by water and sun are just a few of the major topics covered in the Vedas. It began 5000 years ago in Egypt, Germany, India, China, and the United States.

**Question 10**-I'm busy, don't have time for this treatment, as it takes too much of time?

**Answer** -The advantage of nature's cure is that it doesn't take too much of time. You can fast even while working. Other activities like enema take only ten minutes, *Jalneti* takes another ten minutes, hence busy individuals can also perform all the treatments within a limited time frame.

**Question 11**-Is it safe to take Enema at my own?

**Answer** -Yes, it is safe to take enema at home, after practicing couple of times you will do it ease, just follow the instructions mentioned in the chapter.

**Daniel**- Thank you so much, Jack, for your ongoing guidance and clearing my doubts; I will follow the rules of naturopathy and live a healthier life free of medications.

# ENEMIES AND FRIENDS OF YOUR HEALTH

| Enemies | Friends |
|---|---|
| Sugar, Salt | Walk, Exercise |
| Packaged food | Meditation |
| Chemically refined Oil | Keep yourself hydrated |
| Maida | Laugh loud |
| Higher screen time | Think and be positive |
| Negative emotions: Jealous, Anger | Fruits & salads to from 40% of your diet |

# REFERENCES

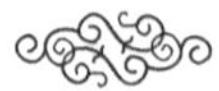

1.Dawas Nature Guide 5$^{th}$ edition by Dr R.S.Dawas

2.Science of Natural Life-Arogya Sewa Prakashan

3.Healthline

www.ingramcontent.com/pod-product-compliance
Lightning Source LLC
Chambersburg PA
CBHW070516160726
48003CB00004B/1593